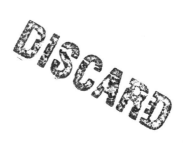

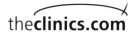

the**clinics**.com

VETERINARY CLINICS

OF NORTH AMERICA

Small Animal Practice

Evidence-Based Veterinary Medicine

GUEST EDITOR
Peggy L. Schmidt, DVM, MS

May 2007 • Volume 37 • Number 3

SAUNDERS

An Imprint of Elsevier, Inc.
PHILADELPHIA LONDON TORONTO MONTREAL SYDNEY TOKYO

W.B. SAUNDERS COMPANY
A Division of Elsevier Inc.

Elsevier, Inc., 1600 John F. Kennedy Blvd., Suite 1800, Philadelphia, PA 19103-2899

http://www.vetsmall.theclinics.com

VETERINARY CLINICS OF NORTH AMERICA:	Volume 37, Number 3
SMALL ANIMAL PRACTICE	ISSN 0195-5616
May 2007	ISBN-13: 978-1-4160-4384-3
Editor: John Vassallo; j.vassallo@elsevier.com	ISBN-10: 1-4160-4384-5

The ideas and opinions expressed in *Veterinary Clinics of North America: Small Animal Practice* do not necessarily reflect those of the Publisher. The Publisher does not assume any responsibility for any injury and/or damage to persons or property arising out of or related to any use of the material contained in this periodical. The reader is advised to check the appropriate medical literature and the product information currently provided by the manufacturer of each drug to be administered to verify the dosage, the method and duration of administration, or contraindications. It is the responsibility of the treating physician or other health care professional, relying on independent experience and knowledge of the patient, to determine drug dosages and the best treatment for the patient. Mention of any product in this issue should not be construed as endorsement by the contributors, editors, or the Publisher of the product or manufacturers' claims.

Veterinary Clinics of North America: Small Animal Practice (ISSN 0195-5616) is published bimonthly (For Post Office use only: volume 36 issue 5 of 6) by Elsevier Inc., 360 Park Avenue South, New York, NY 10010-1710. Months of issue are January, March, May, July, September, and November. Business and Editorial offices: 1600 John F. Kennedy Blvd., Suite 1800, Philadelphia, PA 19103-2899. Customer Service Office: 6277 Sea Harbor Drive, Orlando, FL 32887-4800. Periodicals postage paid at New York, NY and additional mailing offices. Subscription prices are $187.00 per year for US individuals, $297.00 per year for US institutions, $94.00 per year for US students and residents, $248.00 per year for Canadian individuals, $373.00 per year for Canadian institutions, $259.00 per year for international individuals, $373.00 per year for international institutions and $127.00 per year for Canadian and foreign students/residents. To receive student/resident rate, orders must be accompanied by name of affiliated institution, date of term, and the *signature* of program/residency coordinator on institution letterhead. Orders will be billed at individual rate until proof of status is received. Foreign air speed delivery is included in all *Clinics* subscription prices. All prices are subject to change without notice. **POSTMASTER**: Send address changes to *Veterinary Clinics of North America: Small Animal Practice*, Elsevier Periodicals Customer Service, 6277 Sea Harbor Drive, Orlando, FL 32887-4800, USA; phone: 1-800-654-2452 [toll free number for US customers], or (+1)(407) 345-4000 [customers outside US]; fax: (+1)(407) 363-1354; email: usjcs@elsevier.com.

Veterinary Clinics of North America: Small Animal Practice is also published in Japanese by Inter Zoo Publishing Co., Ltd., Aoyama Crystal-Bldg 5F, 3-5-12 Kitaaoyama, Minato-ku, Tokyo 107-0061, Japan.

Reprints: For copies of 100 or more, of articles in this publication, please contact the Commercial Reprints Department, Elsevier Inc., 360 Park Avenue South, New York, New York 10010-1710. Tel. (212) 633-3813 Fax: (212) 462-1935, email: reprints@elsevier.com.

Veterinary Clinics of North America: Small Animal Practice is covered in *Current Contents/Agriculture, Biology and Environmental Sciences, Science Citation Index, ASCA, Index Medicus, Excerpta Medica,* and *BIOSIS.*

Printed in the United States of America.

VETERINARY CLINICS
SMALL ANIMAL PRACTICE

Evidence-Based Veterinary Medicine

GUEST EDITOR

PEGGY L. SCHMIDT, DVM, MS, Diplomate, American College of Veterinary
Preventive Medicine; Assistant Professor, Population Health and Epidemiology,
College of Veterinary Medicine, Western University of Health Sciences, Pomona,
California

CONTRIBUTORS

PETER D. COCKCROFT, MA, MSc, VetMB, DVM&S, Royal College of Veterinary
Surgeons Diplomate in Cattle Health and Production; Diplomate, European
College of Bovine Health Management; Senior Lecturer, Department of
Veterinary Medicine, University of Cambridge, Cambridge, United Kingdom

RICHARD B. EVANS, PhD, Assistant Professor, Veterinary Diagnostic and Production
Animal Medicine, Iowa State University College of Veterinary Medicine, Ames,
Iowa

MARIA A. FAHIE, DVM, MS, Diplomate, American College of Veterinary Surgeons;
Associate Professor, Small Animal Surgery, Western University of Health
Sciences, College of Veterinary Medicine, Pomona; Orange Veterinary Hospital,
Orange, California

KAREN FAUNT, DVM, MS, Senior Director of Medical Support, Banfield, The Pet
Hospital, Portland, Oregon

S. DRU FORRESTER, DVM, MS, Diplomate, American College of Veterinary Internal
Medicine (Small Animal Internal Medicine); Scientific Affairs, Hill's Pet Nutrition,
Topeka, Kansas

MARK A. HOLMES, MA, VetMB, PhD, MRCVS, Senior Lecturer in Preventive
Veterinary Medicine, Department of Veterinary Medicine, University of
Cambridge, Cambridge, United Kingdom

ELIZABETH LUND, DVM, MPH, PhD, Senior Director of Research, DataSavant,
Portland, Oregon

KARI V. LUNSFORD, DVM, Resident and Clinical Instructor in Small Animal Internal
Medicine, Department of Clinical Sciences, College of Veterinary Medicine,
Mississippi State University, Mississippi State, Mississippi

ANDREW J. MACKIN, MVS, DVSc, Associate Professor and Dr. Hugh G. Ward Endowed Chair of Small Animal Medicine, Department of Clinical Sciences, College of Veterinary Medicine, Mississippi State University, Mississippi State, Mississippi

SARAH ANNE MURPHY, MLS, Head, Veterinary Medicine Library, and Assistant Professor, The Ohio State University, Columbus, Ohio

WILL NOVAK, DVM, MBA, Chief Medical Officer and Senior Vice-President of Operations, Banfield, The Pet Hospital, Portland, Oregon

ANNETTE O'CONNOR, BVSc, MVSc, DVSc, Assistant Professor, Veterinary Diagnostic and Production Animal Medicine, Iowa State University College of Veterinary Medicine, Ames, Iowa

STANLEY R. ROBERTSON, DVM, MPH, Associate Professor, College of Veterinary Medicine, Mississippi State University, Mississippi

PHILIP ROUDEBUSH, DVM, Diplomate, American College of Veterinary Internal Medicine (Small Animal Internal Medicine); Scientific Affairs, Hill's Pet Nutrition, Topeka, Kansas

PEGGY L. SCHMIDT, DVM, MS, Diplomate, American College of Veterinary Preventive Medicine; Assistant Professor of Population Health and Epidemiology, College of Veterinary Medicine, Western University of Health Sciences, Pomona, California

DONNA SHETTKO, DVM, Diplomate, American College of Veterinary Surgeons; Associate Professor, Equine Surgery, Western University of Health Sciences, College of Veterinary Medicine, Pomona, California

ROSALIE T. TREVEJO, DVM, MPVM, PhD, Diplomate, American College of Veterinary Preventive Medicine; Assistant Professor of Epidemiology and Veterinary Public Health, College of Veterinary Medicine, Western University of Health Sciences, Pomona, California

VETERINARY CLINICS
SMALL ANIMAL PRACTICE

Evidence-Based Veterinary Medicine

CONTENTS VOLUME 37 • NUMBER 3 • MAY 2007

Over time, evidence-based veterinary medicine (EBVM) should integrate with normal clinical practice. Also, clinical knowledge increases with EBVM, reducing the need for information in one area and allowing veterinarians to explore new areas of specialty or cutting-edge advances in the profession. Textbooks, journals, veterinary conferences, and web sites provide nearly unlimited information about EBVM for the practicing veterinarian to help with the transition to EBVM use in daily practice life. EBVM should continue to change and improve how we, as veterinarians, provide the best available care to our clients and patients.

The ability to translate a clinical problem seen in practice into a focused and well-formed answerable clinical question is one of the hardest steps in practicing evidence-based veterinary medicine (EBVM). Asking answerable clinical questions that relate to your patient is the first evidence-based skill a veterinarian needs to learn, and it forms the cornerstone of the practice of EBVM. Like other clinical skills, the more you practice and work on refining clinical questions, the more precise these questions are and the easier the EBVM process becomes. This article reviews the different aspects of an answerable clinical question, its structure, and how to formulate questions better to get needed answers to clinical problems.

This article offers information regarding selected veterinary information resources, along with basic search strategies for locating clinical evidence within these resources. No one database provides adequate indexing and abstracting to all literature relevant to the veterinary clinical question. An understanding of a database's syntax and field structure is necessary to formulate a functional search strategy and evaluate the outcome of search results. Flexibility when identifying, selecting, and combining search terms is also required to avoid overlimiting a search.

Evaluating the evidence describes the scientific basis of evidence as presented in papers describing the results of clinical research. The types of errors that may lead to misinterpretation of evidence are discussed. This article includes descriptions of the main types of research performed in veterinary clinical research and notes on their advantages and disadvantages.

There is a tremendous amount of medical literature available to the clinician. The challenge is to identify information that is useful and relevant for the patient population of interest. This article provides an overview of important considerations when critically appraising a report, such as selection of the study population, features of the study design used, potential sources of bias, and evaluation of the statistical evidence.

Evidence-based veterinary medicine relies critically on the scientific validity of research. A component of validity is the statistical design and subsequent analysis of data collected during the study. Correct statistical design reduces bias and improves generalizability, and correct analysis leads to appropriate inferences. Inference is the art and science of making correct decisions based on data. Because veterinarians are responsible for the medical care of their patents, it is also their responsibility to understand inferences about treatments presented in papers. This article is designed to assist veterinarians with the interpretation and understanding of statistics presented in papers.

Studies that report the sensitivity and specificity of diagnostic tests are susceptible to flaws that can introduce bias and lead to incorrect estimates. This article uses the quality assessment of diagnostic accuracy studies checklist to describe how to appraise a study reporting diagnostic test comparisons critically. The article also contains a glossary of terms that are useful in discussions about diagnostic tests.

Clinical Reasoning and Decision Analysis
Peter D. Cockcroft

Decision analysis enables outstanding information needs to be correctly identified and ensures that all the options are accurately represented so that appropriate decisions can be made. The aim of this article is to provide an introduction to the use of decision analysis in the practice of evidence-based veterinary medicine. Decision trees using utilities and economic outcomes are presented. The diagnostic process, including the critical appraisal of clinical decision support systems that may be used in this process, is described.

The Power of Practice: Harnessing Patient Outcomes for Clinical Decision Making
Karen Faunt, Elizabeth Lund, and Will Novak

The practice of evidence-based medicine (EBM) relies on the ability of veterinarians to evaluate clinical outcomes. Evaluation of clinical outcomes optimizes the patient care process by transforming what is learned about a population of patients and applying it to an individual patient. Veterinarians' ability to summarize and record relevant information from each pet encounter enables outcomes analysis, thereby transforming clinical data into medical knowledge. This article describes the multiple integrated processes required to evaluate outcomes and practice EBM. As a result of the aggregation and analysis of patient outcomes, knowledge is derived that has the potential to enhance clinical decision making and client communication.

Evidence-Based Management of Feline Lower Urinary Tract Disease
S. Dru Forrester and Philip Roudebush

Many treatments have been recommended for managing cats with feline urinary tract disease (FLUTD). Veterinarians making therapeutic decisions should consider the quality of evidence supporting a recommendation to use (or not use) a particular treatment for cats with FLUTD. Whenever possible, recommendations should be based on results of randomized and well-controlled scientific studies performed in clinical patients with the spontaneously occurring disease of interest. In the absence of such studies, one is left to make the best recommendation possible with consideration of all information, including the quality of the evidence. At this time, additional studies are needed to evaluate evidence for many currently recommended treatments for cats with FLUTD.

VETERINARY CLINICS
SMALL ANIMAL PRACTICE

SEVIER
UNDERS

VETERINARY CLINICS
SMALL ANIMAL PRACTICE

Preface

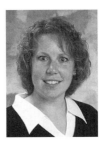

Peggy L. Schmidt, DVM, MS

Guest Editor

T his issue is meant to be a user-friendly guide to the principles and practice of evidence-based veterinary medicine (EBVM) for the practicing veterinarian. It expands on the concepts introduced by Dr. Robert C. Rosenthal in "Evidence-based medicine concepts," the introductory article of the January 2004 *Veterinary Clinics of North America: Small Animal Practice* devoted to Nutraceuticals and Other Biologic Therapies.

Veterinary medicine is not what it used to be. The image of Norman Rockwell's "At the Vet," with the handkerchief-wrapped puppy on his young owner's lap, still permeates the public impression of veterinary practice. This simple image of a puppy with a toothache in a waiting room filled with patients is a poignant reminder of the simplicity of veterinary practice in the past. Today, MRI scans, artificial joints, and organ transplants create a much different image of the profession. Veterinarians provide cutting-edge care for furry four-legged members of the family in much the same way that physicians care for the two-legged family members. Veterinary medical technologies continue to advance at exponential rates. Improvements in current methodologies are rapidly replaced by new diagnostic modalities, therapeutic measures, and prognostic tools.

As a practicing veterinarian, how can we keep up with these rapid changes? It sometimes seems an impossible task. It is not that we lack the capacity to understand veterinary medicine and new technology but that we simply lack the capacity to memorize everything there is to know to succeed. Being able to find the necessary information quickly and efficiently is, and will continue to be, the hallmark of successful veterinarians.

EBVM is a process of clinical decision making that allows veterinarians to find, appraise, and integrate current best evidence with individual clinical

0195-5616/07/$ – see front matter
doi:10.1016/j.cvsm.2007.03.001

expertise, clients' wishes, and patients' needs. It provides tools for identifying information needs, accessing best available evidence, appraising the usefulness and value of the evidence, integrating our knowledge with the patient's needs, and evaluating outcomes of the clinical decision. With practice, EBVM should allow the veterinary clinician to continue to offer the best available medicine as technology and knowledge continue to grow exponentially.

This issue first introduces you to the concept and controversy of EBVM. Individual articles focusing on each of the five steps of EBVM provide in-depth information for how you, as a practicing veterinarian, can adopt EBVM procedures in your daily practice. The three final articles offer examples of evidence-based medicine outcomes for specific questions in small animal practice involving medicine, nutrition, and surgery. The goal of this EBVM issue is to serve as a useful resource for EBVM in any veterinary practice.

Peggy L. Schmidt, DVM, MS
Assistant Professor
Population Health and Epidemiology
College of Veterinary Medicine
Western University of Health Sciences
309 East 2nd Street
Pomona, CA 91766–1854, USA

E-mail address: pschmidt@westernu.edu

Vet Clin Small Anim 37 (2007) 409–417

VETERINARY CLINICS
SMALL ANIMAL PRACTICE

SEVIER
UNDERS

Evidence-Based Veterinary Medicine: Evolution, Revolution, or Repackaging of Veterinary Practice?

Peggy L. Schmidt, DVM, MS

Population Health and Epidemiology, College of Veterinary Medicine, Western University of Health Sciences, 309 East 2nd Street, Pomona, CA 91766–1854, USA

HISTORY OF EVIDENCE-BASED MEDICINE

Human medicine began to recognize the need to substantiate medical decisions with scientific evidence and then to integrate this new knowledge into medical practice as early as the 1970s. In 1972, Cochran [1], a physician for prisoners of war during World War I, published the book, *Effectiveness and Efficiency: Random Reflections on Health Services*. His thoughtful reflections on low morbidity and mortality in the absence of treatment based on current medical recommendations led him to question the effectiveness of the care provided by physicians. Cochran became convinced of the importance of randomized clinical trials (RCTs) to measure efficacy of medical treatments. Soon after publication, other physicians took up the call to improve the medical profession by collecting and cataloging clinical trials. These efforts, led by Dr. Iain Chalmers, evolved over 2 decades into an international nonprofit organization that produces and disseminates up-to-date accurate information about health care interventions—the Cochrane Collaboration [2].

The process of integrating new information and emerging technology into practice was termed *evidence-based medicine* (EBM) in the 1980s by the McMasters' Medical School in Canada. It was not until 1992, however, that the Evidence-Based Medicine Working Group [3] formally proposed EBM as an emerging new paradigm for medical practice, shifting away from medical practice based on observation and experience. Instead, they proposed that medical practice should focus on systematic searches for rigorous scientific evidence. After the boom in EBM-related publications, the term *evidence-based medicine* became an official medical subject heading (MeSH) term in 1997. MeSH terms are a controlled vocabulary of biomedical terms that are used to describe the subject of each journal article in MEDLINE and reflect major topics and categories in medicine and medical terminology. A current search of MEDLINE through PubMed for the term *evidence-based medicine* yields more than 22,000

E-mail address: pschmidt@westernu.edu

journal citations, all published since 1992. Searching for books dealing with EBM concepts reveals thousands of texts and nonfiction titles, emphasizing the past and current recognition of the topic. EBM concepts continue to change and evolve, creating new terms, such as *evidence-based practice* (EBP) and *evidence-based health care* (EBHC), to encompass more than just physician related-medicine but also practice management, public policy, and paraprofessionals, such as nurses and physical therapists.

Evidence-based veterinary medicine (EBVM) may be considered a subspecialty of EBM (after all, we are just another type of medical professional) or a separate individual entity. Determining the origins of EBVM is not easy to accomplish. Using *evidence-based veterinary medicine* as a PubMed search term, we find that the first publication to use the phrase was published in November 2000 [4]. A series of letters appeared in *The Veterinary Record* in the fall of 1998, however, discussing EBM use in the veterinary profession [5–7], and a letter referring to "evidence-based equine medicine" appeared in the *Journal of Equine Veterinary Science* in June 2000 [8]. In this same time frame, veterinary clinical and epidemiology textbooks began to include chapters on EBVM recommendations or techniques.

Regardless of the roots of the term *evidence-based veterinary medicine*, the process of incorporating the EBM principles into the veterinary profession has likely been simmering for decades. More formal promotion and acceptance of EBVM has occurred over the past few years.

The *Handbook of Evidence-Based Veterinary Medicine*, published in 2003, was the first and remains the only textbook dedicated to the use of EBVM [9]. That same year, the *Equine Veterinary Journal* dedicated a special issue to EBM in equine practice [10]. *Veterinary Dermatology* introduced the first in a series of publications on evidence-based veterinary dermatology in the June 2003 issue [11]. In 2004, the College of Veterinary Medicine, Mississippi State University, hosted the first symposium on EBVM, "Using EBM and Outcome Assessment in Veterinary Medicine." Symposium participants used this venue to begin to organize interested veterinarians, which subsequently led to the formation of the Evidence-Based Veterinary Medicine Association [12] during the second symposium on EBVM, "Incorporating Evidence-Based Principles into Veterinary Medicine" in June 2006. General and specialty veterinary conferences and continuing education venues over recent years have also begun to highlight EBVM-related concepts in their seminars and scientific programs.

WHAT IS EVIDENCE-BASED MEDICINE?
Whether using the classic definition by Sackett and colleagues [13], " the conscientious, explicit and judicious use of current best evidence in making decisions abut the care of individual patients," the more current definition by Straus and colleagues [14], "the integration of the best research evidence with our clinical expertise and our patient's unique values and circumstances," or the EBVM definition by Cockcroft and Holmes [9], "a process of lifelong, self-directed problem-based learning," the philosophy remains the same–EBVM is using the best

available evidence and your clinical expertise to make the best clinical decisions for your patients and clients. For more visual learners, a Venn diagram (Fig. 1) may help to illustrate this relation. Ideally, clinical decisions incorporate equal proportions of evidence, clinical expertise, and patient needs or client preferences. In reality, however, as clinicians, we may often weigh each of these important areas differently for each "best clinical decision."

To reach the best decision for each clinical case, the practice of EBVM involves a four- or five-step process.

Steps of Evidence-Based Veterinary Medicine
1. Convert information needs into answerable questions.
2. Efficiently track down the best evidence to answer the question.
3. Critically appraise the evidence for its validity and usefulness.
4. Integrate appraisal results with clinical expertise and patient values.
5. Evaluate outcomes (not included in the four-step process).

Step 1: answerable questions
"Knowing what you don't know" is the basis of Socratic wisdom and the initial phase of the first step of EBVM. As new or unusual cases present diagnostic, therapeutic, or prognostic challenges, veterinarians become aware of key voids in knowledge. Identifying the exact knowledge deficiencies and transforming these information needs into answerable questions may be as challenging as the case before us. Several acronyms exist to help veterinarians create effective questions that aid in efficient searches for answers.

The acronym PICO represents a stepwise process for clearly identifying information needs and serves as a basis for designing an effective clinical question.

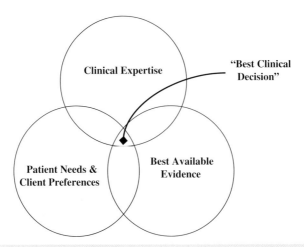

Fig. 1. EBVM is using the best available evidence, your clinical expertise, and specific patient needs and client preferences to reach the best clinical decision for that patient.

P: Patient population. What group do you need information from (eg, species, breed, gender)?

I: Intervention. What is the treatment or procedure do you need or want to take (eg, therapeutics, surgeries, medical procedures, diagnostic tests)?

C: Comparison. What do you want to compare the selected intervention with to assess efficacy (eg, no treatment, past or current standard treatments, medical versus surgical procedures)?

O: Outcomes. What is the effect of the intervention (eg, return to normal function, reduction in severity of clinical signs, increasing expected life span)?

Another acronym gaining popularity is PECOT (population, exposure, comparison, outcome, and time), wherein exposure includes not only interventions but natural exposures to risk factors for disease. As a veterinarian, the importance is not in which acronym you choose to use but that their use increases your ability to identify the information needs for the case at hand efficiently and effectively. See Robertson's article elsewhere in this issue for more in-depth discussion of these principles to help the practicing veterinarian refine clinical questions.

Step 2: finding the evidence

Properly constructed clinical questions ease the search for relevant evidence necessary to make an informed decision. Whether using PICO or PECOT, the words representing each initial become initial keywords in your search. Identifying your keywords is only the beginning, however.

Multiple databases exist in which current literature can be found. One of the most powerful databases is MEDLINE, typically accessed through PubMed. It contains journals for veterinary and human medicine as well as for many allied health professions. Standardized keyword searching is available using MeSH terms. PubMed also includes a "clinical query" function that helps to narrow searches based on your clinical decision (etiology, prognosis, diagnosis, and treatment). Limitations exist for veterinary medicine–related queries. Search filters used by the clinical query feature lack sensitivity or specificity in the veterinary realm [15]. Despite this, PubMed can be a valuable search tool for the practicing veterinarian. Other databases include CAB Direct, AGRICOLA, IVIS, and CONSULTANT. Each database has strengths and weaknesses that you need to be aware of when searching for the necessary evidence. See the article by Murphy elsewhere in this issue for the strengths and weaknesses of these databases.

Despite careful question formulation, database searches may yield few meaningful articles. Keyword choices may be too restrictive (eg, canine) and miss evidence with similar keywords (eg, dog, puppy, bitch, canid). Broadening the scope of the clinical question and using new or revised keywords may identify missing resources. Conversely, if too many resources are retrieved on the initial search, the clinical question should be focused to narrow the scope of retrieved resources. Multiple iterations of clinical questions may be necessary not only for EBVM beginners but for more ardent EBVM users as well.

Step 3: appraising the evidence
Once evidence has been gathered, each article needs to be thoroughly appraised for validity and relevance. All evidence is not created equal, and should therefore be individually evaluated to determine potential significance in decision making. Evidence resources can be applied to a hierarchic "pyramid of evidence" (Fig. 2) to rank the evidence from strongest to weakest. Within each level of evidence, however, individual resources may be evaluated as stronger or weaker after a thorough appraisal. Clinical epidemiology, namely, study design, bias, and statistical inference, provides the framework necessary for critical appraisal of the evidence.

Beyond the strength of evidence and epidemiologic soundness of a study, the results need to be compared to determine if they help to answer the questions posed in step 1 of the EBVM process. The study population should be applicable to the reference population in question—not just in species but the gender, breed, and purpose if possible. Interventions applied in the study must be similar to those in the clinical question. While differences in individual expertise in an intervention, such as surgical skill, may exist between those performing the procedure in the study versus those of the veterinarian searching the literature, the interventions should be judged regardless of level of skill. Comparisons used to determine significance within available literature must be closely related to those identified in the clinical question. Finally, study outcomes must be applicable to the outcome referenced in the clinical question. Proxy variables may represent similar outcomes but should be used with caution. Many studies conclude at ethical end points that may not translate to the end points of interest in actual clinical cases. Caution should be used when extrapolating information

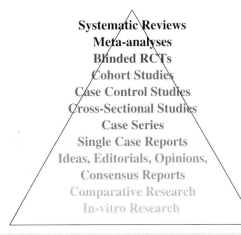

Fig. 2. "Pyramid of evidence" used to rank evidence during critical appraisal of the literature. Resources at the top of the pyramid provide the strongest levels of evidence and progressively become weaker toward the bottom of the pyramid.

from outcomes from differing end points, stages of disease, or "nontypical" routes of infection.

As with developing clinical questions, there are acronyms available to help evaluate literature, such as RAAMbo [16].

R: Who does the study population *represent*? Is it representative of your patient?

A: For intervention studies, how were the animals *allocated* to treatment or exposure groups? Has randomization occurred or, for observational studies, stratification?

A: Are all animals that began the study *accounted* for at the end of the study? If not, do the authors identify what happened to these animals?

M: Were outcome *measurements* in the study evaluated *objectively*, or were evaluators *blinded* to treatment or exposure? This is especially important in observational studies, which often are the highest level of available evidence in veterinary medicine.

Step 4: integrating the evidence

With the information gathered from the best available evidence, a primary plan of action should be in place. But is the client amenable to this plan? Can he or she afford the recommended procedures? Are the best treatment options within the client's ethically, culturally, or religiously acceptable limits? Do you have the knowledge and skills needed to perform the best-evidence procedures? Does your clinic have the necessary technology for the best diagnostic test or process? If not, is the client willing to seek care at a referral center that can provide the service? At this point, we integrate the best available evidence, our clinical expertise, patients needs, and client preferences to decide the best-evidence plan of action.

Internet capabilities have made accessing medical information much easier for veterinarians as well as for our clients. Although most clients lack the necessary skills to question or evaluate the validity of claims made across millions of Web sites, they may present information that they claim refutes your recommendations. As veterinarians we need to be prepared to listen to the client's "evidence" and critically appraise the information. Experience with EBVM and comfort with clinical epidemiology can help to "debunk" many Internet treatment myths and educate clients at the same time.

Step 5: evaluating outcomes

Two outcomes need to be evaluated once the EBVM process nears completion. Foremost, outcomes of the clinical decision need to be evaluated. Did you see the expected results? If not, how did the results differ? Success or failure with attempted diagnostics, treatments, or prognosis can be recorded and used as information in the "clinical expertise" portion of EBVM. With proper record keeping, experiences may also be published as case reports or case series, thereby contributing to the evidentiary portion of EBVM. Significant case numbers, especially with records of outcomes of alternate treatments, may also contribute to the evidentiary portion of EBVM as observational studies. For outcomes to become valuable evidence, standard medical terminology or standard classifications for medical diagnoses should be in place. If not, situations may arise in which apples and oranges are compared because of differing definitions of disease classifications (ie, liver failure versus liver dysfunction).

Evaluation of your individual EBVM outcome or performance is equally important to the evaluation of clinical decision outcomes. This process should include self-evaluation procedures for every step of the EBVM process. Did the clinical question yield the appropriate results? Were too many or too few resources located? Was the critical appraisal process cumbersome? Were the articles internally and externally valid? How did you integrate the client's preferences, patient's needs, and your clinical expertise with the evidence? Were the outcomes of your clinical decision what you expected? Critical self-assessment of the EBVM process allows practitioners to hone their EBVM skills and identify areas for improvement.

EVOLUTION, REVOLUTION, OR REPACKAGING OF VETERINARY PRACTICE?

Confusion about what EBVM is has led to discussion, disillusion, and dissent among veterinarians. Some argue that EBVM is a natural evolutionary progression of clinical medicine occurring after exponential growth in medical and technical knowledge. Others argue that EBVM is a method of practice touted by academics and corporate medicine types who are revolting against the traditional means of veterinary practice. Still others claim that EBVM is merely putting a new face on current veterinary practice rather than a unique new way to practice.

Evolution of Veterinary Medicine

As medical knowledge and technology advance, veterinarians need to evolve their process of accessing new information in the profession in an efficient and effective manner. EBVM formalizes the process of identifying information needs, information gathering, and information processing to help the practicing veterinarian provide the best current practices and procedures for his or her clients and patients. This does not mean that current best evidence has not been used in clinical decisions in the past. Veterinarians have always used evidence to help make clinical decisions, but with the nearly unlimited access to information by means of the Internet, the form and availability of this evidence have changed.

Veterinarians now can access primary literature articles on a much larger scale, allowing new ideas and techniques to play in role in their clinical decisions long before the information is included in clinical textbooks. In the face of evolving public perceptions of the value of companion animals in society, our profession has begun to evolve toward human medicine, with a greater number of specialty areas of practice and diagnostic and treatment modalities rivaling those in human hospitals. It then makes sense that our profession evolves into EBVM practices just as human medicine has done before us and continues to evolve today.

Revolution in Veterinary Medicine

As diagnostic and treatment recommendations for veterinary medicine are increasingly offered by veterinary paraprofessionals or nonveterinary animal "experts," EBVM concepts have been adopted as a means to refute non–scientific-based recommendations. EBMV may have been a grass roots effort to question why veterinarians or other professionals made specific clinical decisions. It provides a framework to agree with or refute those decisions made based on information gathered through pathophysiologic rationale, anecdotal evidence, or "gut feeling." As with many revolutions, there may be initial resistance among the people.

Physicians have met much resistance to the integration of EBM in medical practice. Critics of EBM highlight the lack of physician input in individual cases as a result of standardized care, presumably based on relevant evidence. The heart of this argument is the fallacy that clinical decisions from EBM represent a "one size fits all" approach rather than being tailored to each individual case. This common misconception relates to EBPs or evidence-based guidelines (EBGs), standard procedures based on current best evidence, being interpreted as the only answer for clinical decisions regarding a particular disease etiology, therapy, diagnosis, or prognosis. The application of EBPs and EBGs is a means to standardize treatment options to provide the best medical care rather than a replacement for individual clinical judgment by the clinician. Human medicine has gone a step beyond EBP and EBG to EBHC (also called evidence-based policy making or evidence-based public health), which involves using evidence and the needs and values of a population to make decisions about health care policy. At this point, some say that individual physician preferences may be superseded by the needs of the population and argue that EBHC offsets EBM decisions for the individual patient. Supporters of EBHC maintain that EBHC instead allows for optimal use of valuable medical resources [17]. Veterinary medicine is just beginning to explore this EBHC type of resistance as multisite practices begin to standardize protocols for patients based on evidence-based veterinary guidelines (EBVGs), and the profession is likely to encounter many of the same difficulties that human medicine has faced.

Repackaging of Veterinary Practice

Putting a structured framework around already built clinical decision-making procedures is simply adding new shine to old techniques. Most veterinary professionals do not practice medicine now in the same ways they did on graduation from veterinary school. The drive to excel is inherent in successful veterinarians and compels us to find new techniques and to understand new diseases as they are presented to us. Continuing educations venues, such as conferences, journals, or on-line courses, continue to expand. EBVM and may add consistency to clinical decision-making processes, but the concepts of EBVM are not new to many veterinarians.

SUMMARY

EBVM is not easy for beginners, but then again, do we want to take the easy route when it comes to providing care for our patients? As with any veterinary procedure, practice makes perfect. Adopting EBVM procedures in practice may begin with identifying one pertinent clinical question per day and following though to step 5 and evaluating your performance of the process. Over time, EBVM should integrate with normal clinical practice. Also, clinical knowledge increases with EBVM, reducing the need for information in one area and allowing veterinarians to explore new areas of specialty or cutting-edge advances in the profession. Textbooks, journals, veterinary conferences, and Web sites provide nearly unlimited information about EBVM for the practicing veterinarian to help with the transition to EBVM use in daily practice life. EBVM should continue to change and improve how we, as veterinarians, provide the best available care to our clients and patients.

References

[1] Cochran AL. Effectiveness and efficiency: random reflections on health services. London: RSM Press; 1999.
[2] The Cochrane Collaboration. Available at: http://www.cochrane.org. Accessed February 22, 2007.
[3] Evidence-Based Medicine Working Group. Evidence-based medicine. A new approach to teaching the practice of medicine. J Am Med Assoc 1992;268:2420–5.
[4] Keene BW. Towards evidence-based veterinary medicine. J Vet Intern Med 2000;14(2): 118–9.
[5] Malynicz G. Evidence-based medicine. Vet Rec 1998;143(22):619.
[6] Fogle B. Evidence-based medicine. Vet Rec 1998;143(23):643.
[7] Roper T. Evidence-based medicine. Vet Rec 1998;143(23):644.
[8] Jones WE. Evidence-based equine medicine. J Equine Vet Sci 2000;20(7):415.
[9] Cockcroft PD, Holmes MA. Handbook of evidence-based veterinary medicine. Oxford (UK): Blackwell Publishing; 2003.
[10] Clinical evidence and the evolution of equine evidence-based medicine. Evidence-based medicine special issue. Equine Vet J 2003;35(4):331–422.
[11] Moriello KA. Introducing evidence based clinical reviews in veterinary dermatology. Vet Dermatol 2003;14(3):119–20.
[12] Available at: www.ebvma.org. Accessed February 22, 2007.
[13] Sackett DL, Richardson WS, Rosenberg W, et al. Evidence-based medicine; how to practice and teach EBM. 1st edition. New York: Churchill Livingstone; 1997.
[14] Straus SE, Richardson WS, Glasziou P, et al. Evidence-based medicine; how to practice and teach EBM. 2nd edition. London: Elsevier; 2005.
[15] Murphy SA. Research methodology search filters—are they effective for locating research for evidence-based veterinary medicine in PubMed. J Med Libr Assoc 2003;91(4):484–9.
[16] Jackson R. Can we make appraisal simpler? The GATE tool. In: Conference Report of the 3rd International Conference of Evidence-Based Health Care Teachers & Developers. Taormina (Sicily) 2005. Available at: http://www.ebhc.org/. Accessed February 22, 2007.
[17] Muir Gray JA. Evidence based policy making. BMJ 2004;329:988–9.

Vet Clin Small Anim 37 (2007) 419–431

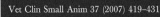

VETERINARY CLINICS
SMALL ANIMAL PRACTICE

SEVIER
JNDERS

Refining the Clinical Question: The First Step in Evidence-Based Veterinary Medicine

Stanley R. Robertson, DVM, MPH

College of Veterinary Medicine, Mississippi State University, PO Box 6100,
MS 39762–6100, USA

Evidence-based medicine (EBM) is the "conscientious, explicit and judicious us of current best evidence in making decisions about individual patients" [1]. It requires integrating best research evidence with our clinical expertise and unique patient circumstances and owner values. Evidence-based veterinary medicine (EBVM) is a practice philosophy and, as defined by Cockcroft and Holmes [2], uses current best evidence in making clinical decisions.

Although many veterinarians believe that they already use the process of evidence-based practice all the time, the observed variation in practice might suggest that this is not always true. Evidence-based practice can be viewed as an attempt to standardize clinical practice. At the same time, however, EBM is not "cookbook" medicine. Because it requires a bottom-up approach that integrates the best external evidence with individual clinical expertise and unique patient circumstances and owner choice, it cannot result in cookbook approaches to individual patient care [3]. External clinical evidence can inform but cannot replace individual clinical expertise, and it is this clinical expertise that decides whether the external evidence applies to the individual patient at all and, if it does, how it should be integrated into the clinical decision for the patient. Similarly, any external guideline must be integrated with individual clinical expertise in deciding whether and how it matches the patient's clinical state, clinical circumstances, and owner's preferences, and then whether it should be applied [4]. The application of EBM may suggest the best approach to a specific clinical problem. It is still up to the veterinarian to determine whether the individual patient is likely to benefit from this approach, however. If your patient is much different from those for whom there is evidence, you may be justified in taking another approach to solve the problem. This decision should be based on sound background and pathophysiologic information.

E-mail address: srobertson@cvm.msstate.edu

0195-5616/07/$ – see front matter
doi:10.1016/j.cvsm.2007.01.002

EVIDENCE-BASED VETERINARY MEDICINE: THE PROCESS

There are five steps involved in the process of EBVM. These steps are sometimes called the educational prescription [5], and they are as follows:

1. Ask an answerable clinical question. Converting the need for information (about diagnosis, prognosis, prevention, therapy, and causation) into an answerable question is the first and most important step in the EBVM process, and it sets the stage for a successful answer to the clinical problem.

   An answerable clinical question has four parts:

   Patient (individual patient, population, or clinical problem of interest)
   Intervention (could be an exposure, diagnostic test, or treatment)
   Comparison (looking at what is better or worse than the intervention)
   Outcome (the clinical outcome of interest to the patient)
   We examine this part (the clinical question) in more detail later in this article.
2. Find the best available evidence to answer that question by searching the veterinary medical literature for studies that are more likely to give the best evidence. This step requires good literature searching skills and knowledge of best information sources (medical informatics).
3. Critically appraise the evidence that is found for its validity (closeness to the truth), relevance (appropriateness), impact (size of the effect), and application (usefulness in our clinical practice). Look for sources of bias that may represent potential flaws in the studies.
4. Apply this evidence by integrating this critical appraisal with your clinical expertise and the patient's specific and unique biology and circumstances.
5. Finally, implement and evaluate the findings in your patient or population, looking at outcomes that are important to you, the patient, and the client.

The ability to translate a clinical problem that is seen in practice into a focused and precise answerable clinical question is one of the hardest steps in practicing EBVM. Asking answerable clinical questions that relate to your patient is the first evidence-based skill a veterinarian needs to learn, and it forms the cornerstone of the practice of EBVM. Like any other clinical skill, the more you practice and work at refining clinical questions, the more precise these questions are likely to be and the easier the EBVM process should become.

REFINING THE CLINICAL QUESTION: BACKGROUND VERSUS FOREGROUND QUESTIONS

Clinical questions can be classified into two basic types: background and foreground questions. Background questions are questions that ask for general knowledge about a disorder. These are questions that have already been answered and are part of our "general knowledge" [4]. Answers to these questions are often found in textbook chapters. Be careful when looking at only answers to background questions, however, because the answers might be incorrect, inaccurate, or out of date. They might not be based on credible evidence. Background questions typically relate to the nature of a disease or disorder or to the usual cause, diagnosis, or treatment of common disorders

[6]. Well-formulated background questions usually have two components (Box 1) [5]:

1. A question root (who, what, when, where, why, or how) with a verb
2. A disorder, test, treatment, pattern of disease, pathophysiology, or other aspect of the disorder

Foreground questions are questions that ask for specific knowledge about managing a patient with a disorder. These questions are usually about recent therapies, diagnostic tests, or current theories of causation of illness. They are usually found at the cutting edge of medicine. The best resources for these questions may include systematic reviews and the primary literature [4]. These questions are at the heart of the practice of EBVM and are designed to provide for this informational need. Well-constructed foreground questions usually have four parts (see Box 1) [7,8]:

1. Patient, population, or problem of interest
2. Main intervention (eg, exposure, treatment, diagnostic test)
3. Comparison intervention to our main intervention
4. Clinical outcome(s) of interest to you, the patient, and the client

---

Box 1: Background versus foreground questions

Background questions
• Ask for general knowledge about a disorder
• Two essential components
  1. A question root (who, what, when, where, why, and how) with a verb
  2. A disorder, test, treatment, or other aspect of the disorder
Examples
What are the causes of renal failure?
What pathophysiologic processes are involved in renal failure?

Foreground questions
• Ask for specific knowledge about managing patients with a specific disorder
• Have four essential components
  1. Patient, population, or problem
  2. Intervention
  3. Comparison of interventions
  4. Clinical outcomes
Example
For canine patients with chronic renal failure attributable to glomerular disease, would adding angiotensin-converting enzyme inhibitors (ie, enalapril) increase survival and quality of life compared with other treatment protocols?

Whether a question is background or foreground depends on one's level of experience with the particular disorder at hand (Fig. 1). When our experience with the condition is limited, as illustrated by point A (like a beginning student), most of our questions (as depicted in Fig. 1 by the vertical dimension) might be related to background knowledge. As our clinical experience and responsibility grow, as illustrated by point B (like a recent graduate), we have increasing proportions of questions related to foreground knowledge for managing patients. Further experience with the condition (like an experienced practitioner or specialist) puts us at point C, where most of the questions are related to foreground knowledge. Notice that the diagonal line is placed to show that we are never too new to learn foreground knowledge or too experienced to have no need for background knowledge.

Do veterinarians need to go through the EBM process for each clinical case they see? When do we want the most current evidence? How often is EBVM needed each day for the average veterinarian? Some of the clinical veterinary work is based on knowledge gained by answering background questions. Nevertheless, there are many situations in which current (and best) evidence is often more helpful. These include questions that are going to have a major impact on our patient. Is the disease fatal; if so, what is the time frame and what are the terminal signs? These are typical questions that a client with a dog that has cancer might want to know about. Other reasons for searching for the best current evidence would include those problems that recur commonly in your practice, those that are of interest to you, or those for which the answer is easily found. This also includes those perplexing cases in which you are confronted with a patient whose problem you cannot solve and for which there is no good background information that would lead you to search for the most current foreground evidence.

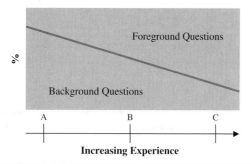

Fig. 1. Relation between background and foreground questions and experience. (*Adapted from* Straus SE, Richardson WS, Glasziou P, et al. Evidence-based medicine: how to practice and teach EBM. 3rd edition. Edinburgh (UK): Churchill Livingstone; 2005. p. 17; with permission.)

CLINICAL QUESTION: THE STRUCTURE OF THE QUESTION

As mentioned previously, the first and most critical part of the evidence-based veterinary process is to ask the right question. The clinical question should have a well-defined structure. This structure should include identifying a patient, intervention, comparison, and outcome [2,4]. These must be clearly stated to search the question actively and efficiently. This model is known by the acronym PICO (patient, intervention, comparison, and outcome), and it has become the standard for stating a searchable and answerable clinical question (Table 1) [8,9].

The patient refers to the patient or population group to which you want to apply the information. First, think about the patient or population that you are dealing with. Try to categorize the patient and identify all its clinical characteristics that influence the problem, are relevant to your practice, and would affect the relevance of research you might find. This may include such things as signalment (age or breed), the primary problem, and the population to which the patient belongs. This would help to identify studies or evidence for similar populations. It may help your search if you can be as specific as possible at this stage; however, keep in mind that if you are too specific with the population, you might have trouble finding any evidence for your patient. If your patient is a 6-year-old male Beagle with chronic weight loss, there might be several studies of current best therapy and management of chronic weight loss in middle-aged dogs but few (if any) studies of chronic weight loss in 6-year-old male Beagles. Asking a question about therapy and management of chronic weight

Table 1		
Components of an answerable clinical question		
Element	Tips	Specific example
Patient (population or problem)	Starting with your patient, ask "How would I describe a group of patients similar to mine?" Balance precision with brevity	"In canine patients older than 10 years of age with chronic renal failure attributable to glomerular nephritis..."
Intervention	Ask "Which main intervention am I considering?" Be specific	"...would the addition of angiotensin-converting enzyme inhibitors to standard chronic renal therapy..."
Comparison of interventions	Ask "What is the main alternative to compare with the intervention?" Again, be specific	"...when compared with standard therapy alone..."
Outcome	Ask "What can I hope to accomplish?" or "What could this exposure really affect?" Again, be specific	"...lead to increased survival time and quality of life"

loss in general is likely to turn up the most evidence. You can then look through these studies to find those applicable to your specific patient.

Intervention is the therapy, prognostic factor, exposure (to potentially harmful process), or diagnostic test that you are considering applying to your specific patient. This could simply be a new drug or diagnostic test. Look at what you want to do for the patient. In therapy, this may be a specific drug or surgical procedure; in diagnosis, it could be a diagnostic test or screening procedure. If the question is about harm or etiology, it may relate to exposure to an environmental agent or examination of the environment to which the animal is exposed. You can also look at what factors might influence the prognosis of the patient, such as age or coexisting disease.

Comparison is comparing the intervention (therapy, etiology, or diagnostic test) with selected interventions by which the intended intervention is measured. A reasonable comparison group would be one that is commonly encountered in clinical practice. Testing a new drug against one that is not used in current practice is not helpful to the practitioner. The comparison group needs to be a real alternative. Some questions that one might ask include the following:

- What is the main alternative to compare with the intervention?
- Are you trying to decide between two drugs or between a drug and no medication?
- Are you trying to decide between two diagnostic tests?

To identify the comparison, a useful approach is to consider what you would do if the intervention was not performed. This may be nothing or a standard care protocol.

The outcome is the end point of interest to you or to your patient and owner. We want to establish what clinical outcome we want to look at. Some things to consider are the following:

- What outcome is important to the patient and the owner?
- What is an appropriate time frame for the response?
- What can you hope to accomplish measure, improve, or affect?
- What are you trying to accomplish for the patient: obtain a cure, prevent deterioration, reduce chronic pain, or increase function?

There is an important distinction to be made between the outcome that is relevant to your patient or population and the outcome measures deployed in the studies. You should spend time working out exactly what outcome is important to you, your patient, and your client as well as the time frame that is appropriate.

Remember that the terms you identify from this process form the basis of your search for evidence and that the clinical question is your guide in assessing its relevance. Again, bear in mind that how specific you are with your question and the terms identified affects the outcome of your search: general terms (eg, *kidney failure*) give you a broad search, whereas more specific terms (eg, *interstitial nephritis*) narrow the search.

One of the benefits of careful and thoughtful question forming is that it makes the search for evidence easier. The well-formed clinical question makes it relatively straightforward to elicit and combine the appropriate terms needed to represent your informational need in the query language of the searching service and searching tools available to you. Once you have formed the clinical question using the PICO structure, you can think about what type of question it is you are asking, and therefore what type of research would provide the best answer.

CATEGORIZING THE TYPE OF CLINICAL QUESTION
Once the question has been created, it is helpful to think about what type of question you are asking. This affects where you look for the answer and what type of research you can expect to provide the answer to your question.

Categories of Different Question Types
There are many different types of questions that can be answered using the evidence-based approach. Many of these questions can be categorized into one of the following groups (Table 2) [2,5]:

Table 2	
Question types for building answerable clinical questions	
Type of question	Type of evidence
Etiology: the causes of disease and their modes of operation	Randomized controlled clinical trial, cohort or case-control study (probably retrospective)
Diagnosis: signs, symptoms, or tests for diagnosing a disorder	Prospective cohort study with good quality validation against "gold standard"
Prognosis: the probable course of disease over time	Prospective cohort study
Therapy: selection of effective treatments that meet your patient's needs and owner values	Randomized controlled clinical trials
Prevention: identification and modification of risk factors to reduce the chance of disease	Randomized controlled clinical trials
Cost-effectiveness: is one intervention more cost-effective than another?	Economic evaluation; analysis of sensible costs against evidence-based outcomes
Quality of life: what will be the quality of life of the patient?	Qualitative study

1. Clinical findings: how to gather and interpret findings from the history and clinical examination
2. Etiology: how to identify causes or risk factors of disease
3. Clinical manifestations of disease: how often and when a disease causes its clinical manifestations and knowing how to use this knowledge to classify a patient's illness
4. Differential diagnosis: when considering the possible causes of a patient's clinical problem, how to rank them in likelihood, seriousness, and treatability
5. Prognosis: how to estimate the patient's likely clinical course over time and anticipate likely complications of the disease
6. Therapy: how to select treatments to offer patients that do more good than harm and that are worth the efforts and costs of using them
7. Control and prevention: how to reduce the chance of disease by identifying and modifying risk factors and how to diagnosis disease early by screening
8. Self-improvement: how to keep up to date and improve clinical and other skills
9. Epidemiologic risk factors
10. Diagnostic process and tests: how to select and interpret diagnostic tests to help confirm or exclude a diagnosis

Knowing what type of question you are asking can also help, to some extent, to narrow down and focus on the kind of research findings needed to help answer the question. Table 2 shows a loose matching of question types to the ideal kinds of research for answering clinical questions. These are just some examples.

To help formulate a well-designed clinical question, you can use a template, such as is illustrated in Table 3. List the concepts and terms for each of the four areas: patient or problem, intervention, comparison of interventions, and clinical outcome. Once you have your terms and concepts listed, you then formulate your clinical question. With practice, this should take only 1 or 2 minutes to complete.

PRIORITIZING THE CLINICAL QUESTIONS

As you go through the evidence-based process, there are often more questions than time to find the answers to them. When this happens, you need to decide which questions to ask. You can consider the following:

- Which question is most important to the patient's well-being and to the owner?
- Which question is most feasible to answer in the time you have available?
- Which question is most interesting to you?

Table 3
Template for formulating well-designed answerable clinical questions

Patient or problem	Intervention	Comparison	Outcome
List concepts here	List concepts here	List concepts here	List concepts here
Your completed clinical question			

Adapted from Heneghan C, Badnoch D. Asking answerable questions. In: Evidence-based medicine toolkit. 2nd edition. Oxford (UK): Blackwell Publishing; 2006. p. 6.

- Which question are you more likely to encounter often in the course of your clinical practice?
- Which question is most likely to benefit your clinical practice?
- Which question has the lowest cost in terms of time but the greatest in terms of clinical cost or benefit?

Prioritizing your clinical questions can help you to make better use of your time and make the evidence-based process more efficient.

CLINICAL QUESTIONS: WHY BOTHER FORMULATING THEM CLEARLY?

Well-formulated clinical questions can help us in clinical practice in several ways [5]:

1. They help us to focus our scarce learning time on the evidence that directly relates to our patients' clinical needs.
2. They help us to focus our scarce learning time on the evidence that directly addresses our specific knowledge needs or the needs of our learners.
3. They can help to suggest high-yield search strategies.
4. They can suggest forms that useful answers might take.
5. They can help us to communicate more clearly with specialists and colleagues when sending or receiving a referral patient.
6. They can help our learners to understand better the content of what we teach while also modeling some adaptive processes for lifelong learning.
7. Our knowledge grows when our questions get answered; in addition, our curiosity is reinforced, and we can become better, faster, and happier clinicians.

In the medical field, research also suggests that clinicians who are taught using this structured approach ask more specific questions [10], undertake more searches [11], use more detailed search methods, and find more precise answers [12,13]. Some groups have begun the implementation and evaluation of question-answering services for medical clinicians with similarly promising initial results [14,15].

TEACHING TO ASK ANSWERABLE CLINICAL QUESTIONS: EDUCATIONAL PRESCRIPTIONS

As mentioned previously, good questions are the backbone of practicing and teaching EBVM, and patients serve as the starting point for both. The challenge to a teacher is to identify questions that are patient based (arising from the clinical problems of a real patient under the learner's care) and learner centered (targeted at the learning needs of the learner) [5]. As we become better skilled at asking these clinical questions, we also become more skilled at teaching others how to do so as well.

As with most other clinical skills, most of us teach question asking best by modeling the formation of good clinical questions in front of our learners. We can also identify our own knowledge gaps and show our learners adaptive ways of responding. Once we have done this by asking a few questions, we can stop and describe explicitly what we did, making note of each of the elements of a good question, whether the questions were background or foreground questions.

The four main steps in teaching learners how to ask good clinical questions are as follows [5]:

1. Recognize: how to identify combinations of a patient's needs and a learner's needs that represent opportunities for the learner to build good questions
2. Select: how to select from the recognized opportunities the one (or few) that best fits the needs of the patient and the learner at that clinical moment
3. Guide: how to guide the learner in transforming knowledge gaps into well-formulated clinical questions
4. Assess: how to assess the learner's performance and skill at asking pertinent answerable clinical questions for practicing EBVM

To recognize potential questions in learners' cases, help them select the "best" questions to focus on, guide them in building the question well, and assess their question-building performance and skill, we need to be proficient at building questions ourselves. We also need the attributes of good clinical teaching, such as good listening skills, enthusiasm, and a willingness to help learners develop to their full potential.

Teaching question-asking skills can be integrated with other clinical skills in the examination room or at cage side, and it does not need to take much additional time. Modeling question formulation often takes less than 1 minute, and coaching learners on developing a question about a patient usually takes 2 to 3 minutes.

Once you and the learners have formulated an important clinical question, how can you keep track of it and follow its progress toward getting a clinically useful answer? One method that has been employed for keeping track is the use of an educational prescription (Fig. 2), which helps teachers and learners in five ways [5]:

1. It specifies the clinical problem that generated the question.
2. It states the question, in all its key elements.
3. It specifies who is responsible for answering that question.
4. It reminds everyone of the deadline for answering the question (taking into account the urgency of the clinical problem that generated it).
5. It reminds everyone of the steps of searching, critically appraising, and ultimately relating the answer back to the patient.

We can also ask our learners to write educational prescriptions for us. This role reversal can help in four ways [5]:

1. The learners must supervise our question-building, making them improve their skills further.
2. The learners can see us admitting our own knowledge gaps; thus, we are practicing what we preach.
3. It can add fun to clinical rounds and sustains group morale.
4. Our learners begin to prepare for their roles as clinical teachers.

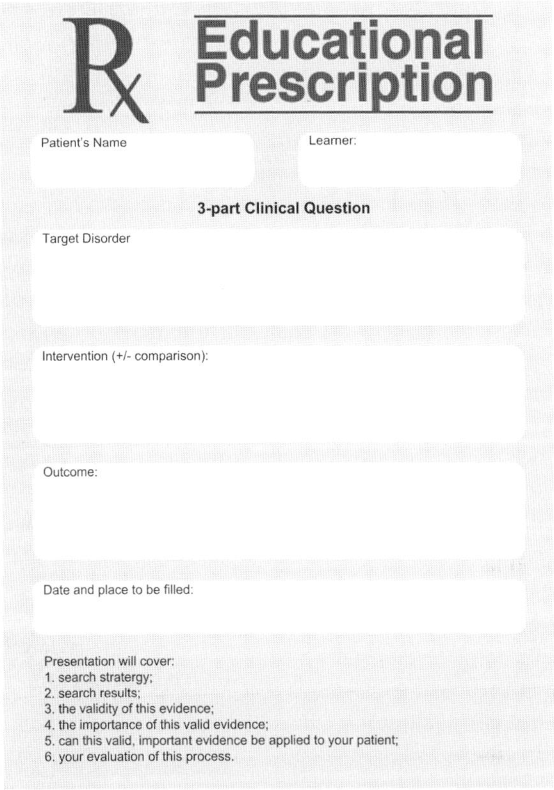

Rx Educational Prescription

Patient's Name

Learner:

3-part Clinical Question

Target Disorder

Intervention (+/- comparison):

Outcome:

Date and place to be filled:

Presentation will cover:
1. search stratergy;
2. search results;
3. the validity of this evidence;
4. the importance of this valid evidence;
5. can this valid, important evidence be applied to your patient;
6. your evaluation of this process.

Fig. 2. Educational prescription form. (*From* Straus SE, Richardson WS, Glasziou P, et al. Evidence-based medicine: how to practice and teach EBM. 3rd edition. Edinburgh (UK): Churchill Livingstone; 2005. p. 26; with permission.)

POTENTIAL PITFALLS IN CONSTRUCTING ANSWERABLE CLINICAL QUESTIONS

There are some potential pitfalls when translating clinical problems into answerable clinical questions that should be considered [2]. Sometimes, the clinical case is just too complicated or there are too many questions generated from the case. In these instances, we might need to prioritize the questions and possibly leave some questions unanswered. We try to get answers to the questions that are most relevant to our particular case and focus on those questions for which we are likely to obtain an answer.

We need to have sufficient background knowledge to formulate good answerable clinical questions. It can be difficult to decide if the breed of the patient is an important factor in the condition in question without knowledge of any breed predisposition. Also, knowledge of any medications or concurrent disease that the patient might have could be important in formulating the clinical question. Background knowledge of such areas as disease processes, pathophysiology, pharmacology, and epidemiology is important in the formulation of well-formed clinical questions. You can seek the opinions of experienced colleagues or specialists in formulating these questions, without necessarily deferring to their opinion as the only answer to the clinical question.

More times than not, we have more questions than we have time to answer. In most veterinary practices, our clients often hope (and expect) a diagnosis, treatment, and prognosis for their animal within the first 15 to 30 minutes of the office examination. This can present a problem for most of us if we are to use evidence-based practices for many of our clinical cases. In the human medical arena, many of the common medical questions are addressed in brief summary form as critically appraised topics (CATs). Currently, there are not collections of CATS in veterinary medicine for clinical practitioners to use. Within a practice or group, however, the work of looking for answers to common clinical question could be shared among individuals in the group and the information collated for practice use. Searching for recently produced evidence and discussing the results can provide an excellent way to make continuing education time enjoyable and productive and enhances lifelong learning.

SUMMARY

Asking answerable clinical questions is the first step in the process of practicing EBVM. It is the cornerstone for the entire process, on which we build by searching for the best available evidence, critically appraising that evidence, applying the evidence to our individual patient, and evaluating the outcome. Time and effort should go into this step so that the other steps are easier and effective. Learning to ask question in a structured format (PICO) helps to ensure clear and precisely written questions. Doing so makes the next step, searching for evidence, easier and more efficient. EBVM is part of an ongoing process of lifelong learning. It should be incorporated into the everyday practice of veterinarians. Asking the right question—an answerable clinical question—is the first step in this process.

References

[1] Sackett DL, Straus SE, Richardson WS, et al. Evidence-based medicine: how to practice and teach EBM. 2nd edition. Edinburg (TX): Churchill Livingston; 2000. p. 1–27.
[2] Cockcroft P, Holmes M. Handbook of evidence-based veterinary medicine. Oxford (UK): Blackwell Publishing; 2003. p. 1–33.
[3] Sackett DL, Rosenberg WM, Gray JAM, et al. Evidence based medicine: what it is and what it isn't. BMJ 1996;312(7023):71–2.
[4] Mayer D. What is evidence-based medicine?. In: Mayer D, editor. Essential evidence-based medicine. Cambridge (MA): Cambridge University Press; 2004. p. 9–16.
[5] Straus SE, Richardson WS, Glasziou P, et al. Evidence-based medicine: how to practice and teach EBM. 3rd edition. Edinburg (TX): Churchill Livingston; 2005. p. 13–30.
[6] Richardson WS. Ask and ye shall retrieve [EBM note]. Evid Based Med 1998;3:100–1.
[7] Oxman AD, Sackett DL, Guyatt GH. Users' guides to the medical literature: I. How to get started. The Evidence-Based Medicine Working Group. JAMA 1993;270(17):2093–5.

[8] Richardson WS, Wilson MC, Nishikawa J, et al. The well-built clinical question: a key to evidence-based decisions [editorial]. ACP J Club 1995;123:A12–3.
[9] Heneghan C, Badnoch D. Asking answerable questions. In: Heneghan C, Badnoch D, editors. Evidence-based medicine toolkit. 2nd edition. Oxford (UK): Blackwell Publishing; 2006. p. 3–6.
[10] Villaneuva EV, Burrows EA, Fennessy PA, et al. Improving question formulation for use in evidence appraisal in a tertiary care setting: a randomized controlled trial. BMC Med Inform Decis Mak 2001;1:4.
[11] Cabell CH, Schardt C, Sanders L, et al. Resident utilization of information technology. J Gen Intern Med 2001;16(12):838–44.
[12] Booth A, O'Rourke AJ, Ford NJ. Structuring the pre-search interview: a useful technique for handling clinical questions. Bull Med Libr Assoc 2000;88(3):239–46.
[13] Rosenberg WM, Deeks J, Lusher A, et al. Improving searching skills and evidence retrieval. J R Coll Physicians Lond 1998;32(6):557–63.
[14] Brassey J, Elwyn G, Price C, et al. Just in time information for clinicians: a questionnaire evaluation of the ATTRACT project. BMJ 2001;322(7285):529–30.
[15] Jerome RN, Gluse NB, Gish KW, et al. Information needs of clinical teams: analysis of questions received by the Clinical Informatics Consult Service. Bull Med Libr Assoc 2001;89(2):177–84.

Vet Clin Small Anim 37 (2007) 433–445

VETERINARY CLINICS
SMALL ANIMAL PRACTICE

SEVIER
UNDERS

Searching for Veterinary Evidence: Strategies and Resources for Locating Clinical Research

Sarah Anne Murphy, MLS

The Ohio State University, 225 Veterinary Medicine Academic Building, 1900 Coffey Road, Columbus, OH 43210, USA

This article continues the evidence-based medicine (EBM) discussion by identifying basic search strategies and information resources required for finding veterinary research. It begins by summarizing selected resources that are useful for locating research applicable to small animal practice. It then outlines basic search strategies for locating evidence within these resources. The article concludes with information on how to obtain articles or books from libraries and other sources and how to use PDAs, RSS feeds, and other tools to acquire and manage information.

OVERVIEW OF SELECT VETERINARY INFORMATION RESOURCES

The usefulness of information is often defined in terms of its relevance and validity in proportion to the amount of time, effort, and resources required to obtain that information [1]. One of the most difficult elements of identifying information for the practice of EBM is the selection of the resource, which depends on the nature of the question; the comprehensiveness of the information needed; the species involved (for veterinarians); and the uniqueness of the disease, diagnosis, or population in question [2]. Because veterinary research is published throughout a broad range of veterinary, agricultural, human medical, and basic science journals, no one database comprehensively provides indexing and abstracting to all literature relevant to the clinical question. Thus, careful searching using a wide variety of information resources is required.

The databases listed here are referred to as "hunting tools" because they are used to pull information once a specific information need has been identified. Tools that push information concerning recent research developments to medical professionals are referred to as "foraging tools" and usually include current awareness publications. Together, hunting and foraging tools complement each other, serving as powerful resources for the identification of valid relevant

E-mail address: murphy.465@osu.edu

0195-5616/07/$ – see front matter
doi:10.1016/j.cvsm.2007.01.003

information directly applicable to patient care. Thus, a medical professional may use a foraging tool to learn of a new development in the field and then relocate the information at a later date with a hunting tool if the new development is not immediately applicable to his or her practice situation. Quality foraging tools (1) comprehensively review the literature for a specific disease, discipline, or specialty; (2) provide a detailed summary of research focused on patient-oriented rather than disease-oriented outcomes; (3) clearly demonstrate assessment of study validity and the level of evidence; and (4) offer specific recommendations, if feasible [1]. The *Compendium on Continuing Education for the Practicing Veterinarian* and *In Practice* offer reviews of the veterinary literature. Although policies requiring authors to follow EBM criteria when preparing reviews for these journals are currently not stated, these journals continue to function as useful foraging tools.

Quality hunting tools offer (1) comprehensive coverage of valid research results; (2) user-friendly searching interfaces; and (3) thesauri to guide the selection of subject terms, key words, or synonyms. Ideally, hunting tools should provide searchable prefiltered reviews of the evidence, such as the *Cochrane Database of Systematic Reviews* does for human medicine, and recommendations based on the assigned level of evidence [1]. Unfortunately, an in-depth resource of comparable quality does not currently exist for veterinary medicine.

The resources discussed here serve mainly as hunting tools to help small animal practitioners identify articles and other sources of veterinary research evidence. Most of these tools provide only summaries of research results. A copy of the actual research article must be obtained for critical appraisal. It is important for a practice to maintain a small collection of core veterinary research and review journals, along with EBM-oriented reference texts, and to have procedures in place for obtaining articles, conference proceedings, book chapters, or reports not held locally. Although this list is by no means comprehensive, the tools discussed are the most useful for identifying current evidence-based veterinary research.

CAB Direct

A product of CAB International, a not-for-profit publisher of life sciences books, databases, and primary journals, CAB Direct offers the most comprehensive indexing and abstracting of the veterinary literature [3]. If purchased in conjunction with the CAB Archive, the database includes citations for journals, conference proceedings, books, book chapters, theses, dissertations, annual reports, patents, and international standards from 1910 to the present. As the online equivalent of the *Index Veterinarius* and *Veterinary Bulletin*, its strength is its international coverage of the animal health literature. Complementary subjects covered within the database include animal breeding and genetics, animal nutrition, and aquaculture.

CAB Direct offers a detailed hierarchical thesaurus, which assists searchers with refining searches by suggesting broader and narrower terms. An option to limit by geographic terms is also available so that searchers may identify research articles addressing certain concerns in specific areas or regions of the world.

A subscription is required to access CAB Direct. For the retrieval of relevant veterinary research evidence, however, CAB Direct is worth the investment, because time-saving value-added features allow the small animal practitioner to export citations for personal use directly to e-mail or to reference management software. Individual subscriptions may be obtained through CAB International's VetMed Resource product for veterinarians [4].

Pubmed (MEDLINE)*

As the premiere biomedical sciences database of the US National Library of Medicine, PubMed provides free access to more than 13 million citations and abstracts from more than 4800 scientific journals in medicine, nursing, dentistry, veterinary medicine, health care systems, the preclinical sciences, and other additional life sciences [5]. Although PubMed's free status is attractive, its coverage of veterinary medicine is limited to veterinary science in relation to human health. Approximately 80 major veterinary journals are indexed in PubMed, including the *Journal of the American Veterinary Medical Association*, all four editions of the *Veterinary Clinics of North America*, the *Journal of the American Animal Hospital Association*, and the *Journal of Small Animal Practice*. Other important veterinary titles, however, such as *Compendium on Continuing Education for the Practicing Veterinarian,* and *Equine Veterinary Education* are not covered. Further, unlike CAB Direct, PubMed provides indexing and abstracting for the journal literature only.

PubMed operates on Entrez, the National Center for Biotechnology Information's (NCBI's) text-based search and retrieval system. The database includes MEDLINE, OLDMEDLINE, and in-process and publisher-supplied citations. Other Entrez-supported databases, such as Professor Frank Nicholas' *Online Mendelian Inheritance in Animals*, the NCBI's *Taxonomy Database*, and *PubMed Central* (the National Library of Medicine's digital archive of free life sciences journals), may be accessed through PubMed, providing additional types of important non–citation-based information.

Updated daily, PubMed covers journal literature back to the early 1950s. The database's strength is that it is indexed using medical subject heading (MeSH) terms, a controlled vocabulary. All queries directly entered into the PubMed search box are first matched to a MeSH translation table, a journals translation table, and, finally, an author index [6]. The benefit of this behind-the-scenes programming is that the database automatically maps the various key words you enter into the PubMed search box to standardized subject headings. This reduces the need to enter different terminology for the same concepts. A basic understanding of the database architecture is still required, however, for effective interpretation and evaluation of search results.

---

*Animated tutorials demonstrating how to search the database for human information are available at http://www.nlm.nih.gov/bsd/disted/pubmed.html.

AGRICOLA

AGRICOLA is a free public access database of books and article citations compiled by the US National Agriculture Library [7]. Covering agriculture and related disciplines, AGRICOLA selectively indexes the veterinary literature, and therefore is not as comprehensive in coverage as CAB Direct or PubMed. AGRICOLA, however, can be useful for locating veterinary information pertaining to production animals and animal welfare in particular. It is also an excellent source for locating US Department of Agriculture (USDA) publications. The database is designed to be searched using free-text key words.

Consultant

A product of Dr. Maurice White at Cornell University, Consultant functions as a diagnostic support tool and a continuously updated veterinary textbook [8]. Designed with the veterinary practitioner in mind and updated daily, the database links approximately 500 clinical signs and symptoms to more than 7000 possible diagnoses or disease conditions. It may be searched by the clinical signs observed to determine a probable cause for a diagnosis or by a disease itself. A description is provided for each disease covered in the Consultant database, along with a listing of the species it affects, possible signs, and a list of article and web site references.

International Veterinary Information Service

With an international editorial board consisting of veterinarians and veterinary researchers steering the project and a veterinary librarian advisory board in place to advise the editorial board on means to enhance the value of its Web site, the International Veterinary Information Service (IVIS) provides free access to electronic books, conference proceedings, short courses, continuing education, and other information products in multiple languages for veterinarians, veterinary students, and animal health professionals worldwide [9]. In addition to offering full-text books, the library section of the Web site provides a table of preset journal and species limits for PubMed, assisting searchers with limiting searches to small animals, horses, ruminants, and pigs. Although free, registration is required to use this Web site.

Veterinary Information Network

A subscription-based service, the strength of the Veterinary Information Network (VIN) is its message boards, where practicing veterinarians may post a question and seek answers from VIN-employed veterinarians or other members of the VIN community [10]. VIN also provides continuing education (CE) opportunities, rounds discussions, newsletters, and a forum for veterinary support staff personnel.

SEARCH STRATEGIES, HEURISTICS, AND MECHANICS FOR LOCATING VETERINARY INFORMATION

Search strategies encompass the overarching plan or approach to the search for information. Search heuristics represent the steps taken to advance search objectives or modify a particular search strategy as the search develops [11]. Again, because veterinary research is scattered throughout veterinary, agricultural, human medical, and basic science journals, no one database comprehensively indexes and abstracts all literature that may provide a relevant answer to the clinical question. Selection of resource(s) depends on the search subject and the depth or comprehensiveness of information required. Because search interfaces vary widely among vendors and platforms, familiarizing oneself with the structure of at least two or three databases is recommended; this permits an understanding of the database syntax and field structure for each resource. This also enables the small animal practitioner to refine search strategies and to search more efficiently as searching skills improve. It is important to understand that database searching is as much an art as it is a science and that the search outcome should always be of primary interest.

The first step in creating an effective search strategy involves formulating the clinical question. By developing a patient, intervention, comparison, and outcome (PICO) statement, as outlined in the article on refining the clinical question by Robertson in this issue, major concepts for the search may be identified and a functional search strategy can be developed by determining how these concepts relate to one another. Concepts may be represented by one word or a series of words.

For example, suppose an information need regarding treatment of fungal keratitis in cats is developed using a PICO statement. One strategy is to use the concepts from the PICO statement to create building blocks to identify similar or related terms for each concept and then to link the concepts together using the Boolean operators "AND," "OR," or "NOT" (Fig. 1).[†] An advantage of setting a search up this way is that the strategy can easily be modified to search more than one database.

In Fig. 1, synonyms are listed in blocks 1 and 2 for the population/patient/problem concepts "fungal keratitis" and "cats." Note that in block 1, the word "keratomycosis" is listed as a synonym for fungal keratitis. If you search the CAB Direct Thesaurus using the word "keratitis," *keratomycosis* is listed as the preferred term under mycotic keratitis (Fig. 2). Thesauri are powerful tools for identifying synonyms, related terms, broader terms, and narrower terms to use for increasing the recall or precision of a search. PubMed's thesaurus is known as the MeSH Database. A search on fungal keratitis, keratomycosis, and mycotic keratitis using the MeSH Database does not return relevant hits. If you search the MeSH Database, however, using the term *eye infections*, the narrower term *eye infections, fungal* appears. Careful examination of the MeSH record for "eye infections, fungal" reveals that "oculomycosis," "mycosis, ocular," "ocular infection, fungal," and 20 other variations are automatically mapped to this subject heading (Fig. 3). This illustrates the benefits of flexibility in thought and action when formulating and executing a search

---

[†]For a brief review of Boolean operators, an online tutorial is available at net.TUTOR (see "Searching 101" at http://liblearn.osu.edu/tutor/les4/).

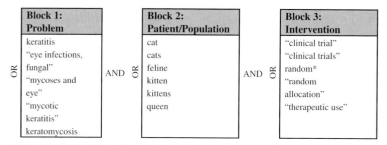

Block 1: Problem		Block 2: Patient/Population		Block 3: Intervention
keratitis "eye infections, OR fungal" "mycoses and eye" "mycotic keratitis" keratomycosis	AND OR	cat cats feline kitten kittens queen	AND OR	"clinical trial" "clinical trials" random* "random allocation" "therapeutic use"

Fig. 1. Building Blocks.

strategy. Sometimes, the initial search terms selected do not yield desired results. The initial search results, however, may provide valuable clues to help improve the search. Note that by searching one term in the CAB Thesaurus and MeSH Database, additional synonyms or related terms were identified for the search. Information scientists call this "pearl growing," a technique that is particularly useful when you need to find specific information in a subject area but have little knowledge of or experience with the vocabulary of that subject area. Just as a pearl grows by adding layers, recall for a search can be improved, layer by layer, by adding synonyms and related terms to a search [11]. The technique can also be used as a search strategy if you have one good article. Using your one good article, you can identify other quality articles

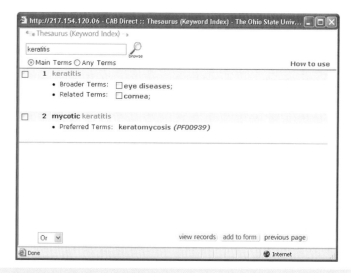

Fig. 2. "Keratitis" in CAB Direct Thesaurus.

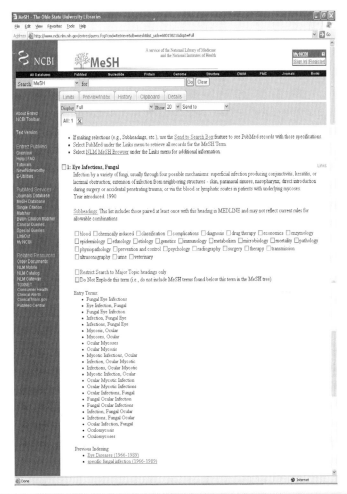

Fig. 3. "Eye Infections, Fungal" in MeSH Database.

by examining how the good article was indexed in a database and then use the indexing terms for the good article to find other related articles.

In block 3 of Fig. 1, the terms *clinical trial*, *clinical trials*, *random**, *random allocation*, and *therapeutic use* are listed under therapy. The quotations indicate that these are phrases, meaning the database should identify the two words in sequence. In some databases, it is acceptable to identify phrases using quotes. In others, individual terms must be linked together using the Boolean operator AND. The asterisk after the word "random" is a truncation symbol, which is used to search for plurals and other variations of a word root. The terms listed in block 3 of Fig. 1 are from a standard EBM filter promoted by Haynes and colleagues [12,13] for identifying clinical research evidence related to treatment in PubMed.[‡] Although this filter does suggest good search terms to identify high-quality evidence for therapy decisions, without modification, it does not translate well for locating veterinary evidence, especially in other databases, such as CAB Direct [14,15]. In most cases, the filter is going to return a search with limited, misleading, or no results, because the evidence hierarchy for veterinary medicine includes less established research methodologies. This topic is addressed in further detail in another article in this issue. When the recall of a search needs to be limited or reduced, however, it is useful to employ search heuristics to modify the search by adding or removing selected terms as necessary to improve the precision of the search.

Recall represents the number of relevant documents retrieved in proportion to the total number of relevant documents in a database. A search with good recall should have high sensitivity, returning a broad range of results. Precision represents the number of relevant documents retrieved in proportion to the total number of documents retrieved. A search with good precision should retrieve a narrower set of results. Execution of a search strategy depends on the database selected and the recall and precision desired for the search. Using the building blocks strategy, in situations in which it is believed that using all the identified concepts is likely to result in the retrieval of few or no articles, start by searching the most specific concept first, such as block 1 in Fig. 1. Assess the output, and then add concepts with broader search terms to the search to increase recall, or delete broader more ambiguous terms while adding narrower concepts to increase precision. In many cases, a search for veterinary information can begin by identifying the problem of interest and then limiting by the species. Thus, we can begin with the terms listed in block 1 and limit our results using the terms listed in block 2.

As mentioned previously in this article, PubMed has been programmed to map concepts to standardized subject headings and to insert appropriate search fields and Boolean terminology for you. Thus, if the words "fungal keratitis cats" are entered directly into the PubMed search box, relevant results are returned. A basic understanding of search strategies and database architecture, however, is still necessary, because PubMed sometimes fails to interpret the query as envisioned by the searcher. Thus, check the details tab after every PubMed search to see how the database constructed the search (Fig. 4). Additional limits and search terms can be added to or deleted from the search using this feature to modify the search strategy as appropriate. A basic knowledge of MeSH headings, however, is still necessary. For example, if the same search is run using a slightly different strategy by entering the MeSH headings for "eye infections, fungal" AND "cats," relevant results are also returned, but these

---

[‡]Recent research indicates that the PubMed publication type limit for clinical trial is effective for delivering sensitive search results in PubMed [12]. Additional research methodology search filters for diagnosis, etiology, prognosis, and clinical prediction guides are available at http://www.ncbi.nlm.nih.gov/entrez/query/static/clinicaltable.html.

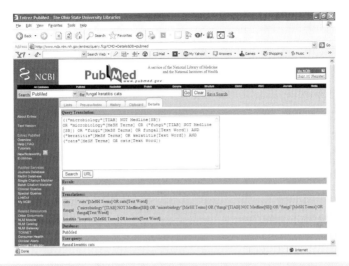

Fig. 4. Details of PubMed Search Using the Keywords "fungal keratitis cats."

results are different from those of the previous search. A veterinary subheading (ie, "eye infections, fungal/veterinary" [MeSH]), however, may be used with MeSH terms to limit searches to veterinary applications.

In CAB Direct, terms are not automatically mapped to standardized subject headings, reinforcing the need to familiarize yourself with database syntax, mechanics, and overall architecture. To construct a key word search for this database, the Boolean operators AND and OR would need to be used to link the terms in building block 1. For example, if we constructed this search using the advanced search feature of CAB Direct, we would type the words "mycotic and keratitis" or "fungal and eye and infection" or "mycoses and eye" in the first search line while selecting all fields from the pull-down menu (Fig. 5). In the second search line, we would select the Boolean operator OR from the pull-down menu and then type in "keratomycosis" and select the subject term field from the pull-down menu, because we have already identified this word as an indexing term in CAB Direct. In the third search line, we would select the Boolean operator AND from the pull-down menu and then type in terms from building block 2 for cats: *cat* or *cats* or *feline* or *kitten** or *queen*. If we realize that further limits are needed after we run the initial search, we can run a search within the search results using selected terms from building block 3, such as *clinical* and *trial*, with a limit for publication year (Fig. 6).

A danger in the formulation of any search strategy is inflexibility in selection of search terms. The searcher must be willing to brainstorm, identifying synonyms or broader search terms along with different combinations of concepts, to

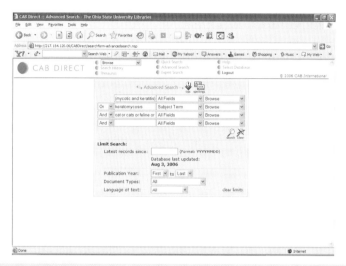

Fig. 5. Search for "fungal keratitis" records in CAB Direct.

avoid overlimiting a search to the point where no relevant results are returned. This is particularly important in databases other than PubMed, which do not automatically map search terms to subject headings. "A mindless faith in controlled vocabularies," however, as illustrated by the PubMed example provided previously, "is not always justified" [11].

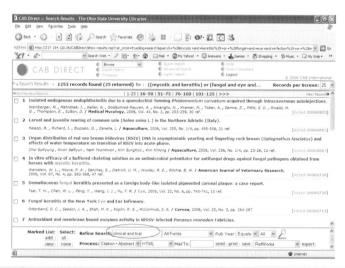

Fig. 6. Search with CAB Direct Search Results Using terms *clinical* and *trial*.

LIBRARIES, RSS FEEDS, PDAS, AND OTHER TOOLS FOR LOCATING AND ACQUIRING INFORMATION

Inadequate access to information at the point of care is often cited as one of the most significant barriers to the practice of EBM [16]. Indeed, finding time to search for and analyze clinical research evidence is challenging. Fortunately, recent advances in information technology can assist medical professionals with identifying research evidence when it is relevant and directly applicable to patient care. For example, Cornell University's *Consultant* database, with its simple design, can easily be searched using a PDA or "smart phone" with Internet access. Thus, veterinary professionals have a free diagnostic decision support tool available to them that they can essentially carry around in their pocket. A search on keratitis using this source returns a set of possible diagnoses that includes a description of fungal keratitis and a list of recent citations related to the disorder. PubMed also functions well on PDAs, using a reformatted text-based interface known as *PubMed for Handhelds* [17].

Many databases are also now enabling individuals to establish an RSS feed to notify them when a new article is indexed on a specific subject. RSS is a Web standard that allows your computer to browse the Web looking for specific information for you and then to deliver the information to you where and when you want it. To read RSS feeds, an RSS reader is required. Some Web browsers, such as Mozilla, have an RSS reader built directly into their software. Many other independent RSS readers are available for free download on-line.

In PubMed, an RSS feed may be established by first running a search on the topic to monitor and then selecting "RSS feed" from the "send to" pull-down menu at the top of the screen (Fig. 7). On the next screen, click on "create feed" and then click on the orange XML icon that appears. In the new window that

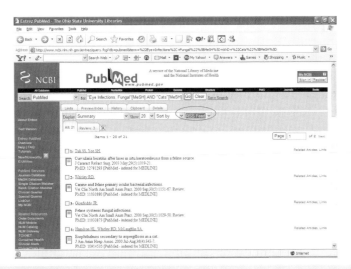

Fig. 7. Setting up RSS feeds in PubMed.

opens, copy the uniform resource locator (URL) in the browser address box and paste it into your RSS reader. After establishing an RSS feed, when a new article is indexed on this topic, you are notified by means of your RSS reader. PubMed also has a service known as "My NCBI" (previously called "Cubby"), where individuals may save searches and receive an e-mail alert when new content matching the search terms is added.

Finally, although it is important to maintain a small collection of information sources for local use, it is also important to have procedures in place for obtaining information resources not available locally through alternative sources. Most publishers offer reprints of the articles they publish for a fee through their Web sites. A small number of veterinary journals, including the *Canadian Journal of Veterinary Research, Canadian Veterinary Journal,* and *BMC Veterinary Research,* now operate on an open-access model, making their articles freely available through Web sites, such as PubMed Central, immediately or after a 3- to 6-month embargo [18]. Unlike in the United Kingdom, where the RCVS Trust operates, a full-service membership-supported veterinary medical library is not available in the United States. Many veterinary medical schools in the United States, however, provide library outreach services to alumni and local veterinary professionals. Although policies for these services differ among schools, document delivery and library reference assistance is usually available. A chart indicating the specific services provided by each US veterinary school library is published in the annual American Veterinary Medical Association (AVMA) membership directory [19]. Although library fees for document delivery requests are common, these fees are sometimes lower than the fees charged by the publisher, because the library may subsidize a portion of their service for the small animal practitioner. Most libraries also have the technology to deliver article requests directly to the desktop as an electronic PDF file.

SUMMARY

This article offers information regarding selected veterinary information resources, along with basic search strategies for locating clinical evidence within these resources. No one database provides adequate indexing and abstracting to all literature relevant to the veterinary clinical question. An understanding of a database's syntax and field structure is necessary to formulate a functional search strategy and evaluate the outcome of search results. Flexibility when identifying, selecting, and combining search terms is also required to avoid overlimiting a search.

Because the hierarchy of veterinary research evidence encompasses a broader range of acceptable research methodologies, the EBM search filters promoted by Haynes and colleagues [12] for locating clinical evidence for human medicine do not translate well to the veterinary environment. Other articles in this issue discuss which types of veterinary research methodologies to be looking for when searching for clinical evidence, how to prioritize them, and how to analyze studies for application to clinical practice once they have been identified.

Acknowledgments

The author gratefully acknowledges the following individuals for their assistance in the preparation of this article: Carol Powell, Instruction Librarian, John A. Prior Health Sciences Library, The Ohio State University; Ana Ugaz, Clinical Librarian, Medical Sciences Library, Texas A&M University; Katherine Anderson, Specialized Services Librarian, J. Otto Lottes Health Sciences Library, University of Missouri-Columbia; and Sarah McCord, Electronic Resources Librarian, Health Sciences Library, Washington State University.

References

[1] Slawson DC, Shaughnessy AF. Teaching evidence-based medicine: should we be teaching information management instead? Acad Med 2005;80:685–9.

[2] Koonce TY, Giuse NB, Todd P. Evidence-based databases versus primary medical literature: an in-house investigation on their optimal use. J Med Libr Assoc 2004;92:407–11.

[3] CAB International. CAB Direct. Available at: http://www.cabdirect.org. Accessed February 22, 2007.

[4] CAB International. VetMed Resource. Available at: http://www.vetmedresource.org. Accessed February 22, 2007.

[5] National Center for Biotechnology Information. National Library of Medicine. National Institutes of Health. Available at: http://pubmed.gov. Accessed February 22, 2007.

[6] National Center for Biotechnology Information. National Library of Medicine. National Institutes of Health. How PubMed works: automatic term mapping. Available at: http://www.ncbi.nlm.nih.gov/books/bv.fcgi?rid=helppubmed.section.pubmedhelp. Appendices#pubmedhelp.How_PubMed_works_aut. Accessed April 26, 2006.

[7] National Agriculture Library. United States Department of Agriculture. Agricola. Available at: http://agricola.nal.usda.gov/. Accessed February 22, 2007.

[8] White, Maurice E, consultant. Available at: http://www.vet.cornell.edu/consultant/consult.asp. Accessed February 22, 2007.

[9] International Veterinary Information Service. Available at: http://www.ivis.org. Accessed February 22, 2007.

[10] Veterinary Information Network, Inc. Available at: http://www.vin.com/. Accessed February 22, 2007.

[11] Harter SP. Search strategies and heuristics. In: Online information retrieval: concepts, principles, and techniques. Orlando (FL): Academic Press; 1986. p. 170–204.

[12] Haynes RB. Clinical queries using research methodology filters. Available at: http://www.ncbi.nlm.nih.gov/entrez/query/static/clinicaltable.html. Accessed April 26, 2006.

[13] Glanville JM, Lefebvre C, Miles JN, et al. How to identify randomized controlled trials in MEDLINE: ten years on. J Med Libr Assoc 2006;94:130–6.

[14] Murphy SA. Research methodology search filters: are they effective for locating research for evidence-based veterinary medicine in PubMed? J Med Libr Assoc 2003;91:484–9.

[15] Murphy SA. Applying methodological search filters to CAB abstracts to identify research for evidence-based veterinary medicine. J Med Libr Assoc 2002;90:406–10.

[16] Green ML, Ciampi MA, Ellis PJ. Residents' medical information needs in clinic: are they being met? Am J Med 2000;109:218–23.

[17] National Library of Medicine. PubMed for handhelds. Available at: http://pubmedhh.nlm.nih.gov/nlm/. Accessed April 26, 2006.

[18] PubMed Central. Available at: http://www.pubmedcentral.nih.gov/. Accessed April 26, 2006.

[19] American Veterinary Medical Association. AVMA membership directory and resource manual. Schaumburg (IL): The Association; 2006. p. 325–32.

Vet Clin Small Anim 37 (2007) 447–462

VETERINARY CLINICS
SMALL ANIMAL PRACTICE

Evaluation of the Evidence

Mark A. Holmes, MA, VetMB, PhD, MRCVS

Department of Veterinary Medicine, University of Cambridge, Madingley Road,
Cambridge CB3 0ES, UK

In attempting to provide the best veterinary care for our patients, we make a series of decisions, which, unless we are completely irrational, are made on the basis of evidence. To provide the best possible decisions, we need to be able to rank this evidence. Common sense tells me that my lecture notes from some 20 years ago are likely to yield poorer evidence than a recent issue of *Veterinary Clinics of North America*. The age of the information, or the eminence of the authors, seems a haphazard way of arriving at the quality of the evidence as it applies to my particular patient, however, and evidence-based veterinary medicine (EBVM) has emerged as a more methodical and systematic approach to establishing the best evidence for a clinical decision.

We need to consider the scientific basis by which information or evidence supporting the choice of particular clinical interventions is based. Science, or the scientific process, is a search for truth and acknowledges our natural human failings. There are three main areas in which one is likely to be misled: these are false assumptions of knowledge, bias, and chance.

Although clients (and veterinarians) crave certainty, we know that our knowledge is finite and that every incidence of a disease is a unique entity. Early in our clinical careers, we discover that a previously held belief about a treatment or a diagnosis turned out to be wrong. Before the 1990s, it was widely believed that infants should be placed face down to sleep and that those sleeping on their backs were at a greater risk of choking on their vomit if they were sick. A result of a meta-analysis of many studies of sudden infant death syndrome (SIDS) revealed that the incidence of SIDS was lower in infants placed on their backs to sleep. After a public health campaign in the 1990s, the incidence of SIDS in the United States was reduced by more than 40% (from 1.4 to 0.8 deaths per 1000 births) [1]. Here is a clear example of how a rationally held belief was actually wrong and led to avoidable infant deaths. We can never be certain about the veracity of our knowledge and should make every attempt to find and evaluate new evidence to reduce that uncertainty.

There are many forms of bias that cloud our judgment or perception. In Fig. 1, there is a picture of two tables. The one on the left looks longer and

E-mail address: mah1@cam.ac.uk

0195-5616/07/$ – see front matter
doi:10.1016/j.cvsm.2007.01.004

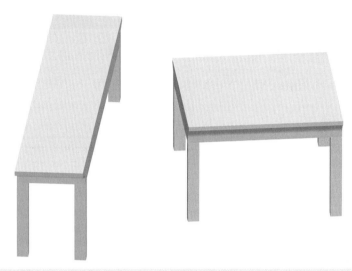

Fig. 1. Example of an optical illusion in which two tables seem to be of different size. Measurement of the dimensions of the two tabletops as they appear in the illustration shows that they are identical.

narrower than the one on the right, but if you measure the dimensions of the two tabletops, you discover that they are identical. We cannot even trust the evidence of our own eyes. When clinical research is performed, it is only natural for the investigators to want to detect a substantial treatment effect or discriminatory power of a clinical test. This inevitably leads to conscious or unconscious bias in the measurement or presentation of results if researchers do not take steps to avoid this bias. If clinical research is performed using purebred laboratory animals, there may also be confounding factors associated with the breed or husbandry of these animals that render the results of such research inapplicable to our patients.

The final major source of error is attributable to chance and our ability to assess risk. Hope and fear obscure our ability to estimate risk properly. The success of the gambling industry is powerful evidence of this. When a gambler has a run of luck, it is only human to try and ascribe this to anything other than pure chance. We have good recall of our spectacular successes and failures among our clinical cases, but we tend to forget about the myriad of run-of-the-mill cases that form most of our caseload. The only weapon we have in our armory to deal with this is the use of statistics. Basic numeracy and an understanding of the main sources of statistical errors are essential if we are to be able to evaluate the results of clinical research as described in the article on statistics and evidence-based veterinary medicine by Evans and O'Connor elsewhere in this issue.

Having acknowledged that we might be wrong, we need to appreciate that we can look at evidence from a variety of sources and judge its quality. The best sources of evidence are those that result from a scientific experiment.

SCIENTIFIC EVIDENCE

All that is meant by "scientific" is that an empirically testable (ie, something that can be observed) question was asked. In clinical research, this is normally something like, "Is treatment A better than treatment B?" or "Is diagnostic test X better than diagnostic test Y?" If it is not possible to answer the question with an empiric test, the theory that a particular treatment is better than another has, to all intents and purposes in clinical medicine, no scientific basis. The theory held is a nonscientific belief. A test is just an observation, and an experiment is a set of arrangements put in place to permit the observation to be made.

The essence of science is the balance between skepticism and open-mindedness. On the one hand, we are constantly asking ourselves, "Could there be an alternative explanation for what we have observed?" Conversely, we should be prepared to accept that any scientifically testable theory could be true until it has been subjected to a test and seen to fail.

RANKING THE EVIDENCE

The hierarchy of evidence is a broad categorization of sources, highlighting those that are the most likely to produce the best evidence. Each piece of evidence arising from clinical research that provides evidence has some intrinsic qualities that enable us to anticipate its relative quality. A well-conducted randomized controlled trial (RCT) provides better evidence than an uncontrolled case series; an RCT with more animals in each treatment group provides stronger evidence when compared with a similar trial with fewer subjects. It must be appreciated that the intrinsic qualities of a particular study design may be rendered useless if there is a major flaw in the way the study is conducted. An important aspect in the evaluation of the results of clinical research as evidence is the critical appraisal of the research paper, which is described by Trevejo elsewhere in this issue. The hierarchy of evidence is often represented as a pyramid (Fig. 2). Although it may be optimistic to expect there to be a substantial "pyramid of evidence" for every veterinary clinical question, an understanding of the merits of different types of study is important to enable us to begin the appraisal process.

RESEARCH PAPERS

The scientific papers we find when we search literature databases fall into three main categories. At the top of the pyramid of evidence are papers describing the results of research synthesis. Although research synthesis has been used to represent many activities, in the scientific community, it is a systematic process of summarizing research that has evolved over the past few decades into a science of its own and typically results in the production of systematic reviews and meta-analyses. The second category of literature are those papers that describe the results from the comparison of groups of animals, usually an experimental group and a control group (explanatory studies). These are often tests of an intervention or a diagnostic test. The final category consists of those papers reporting descriptive studies. Descriptive studies are designed to record

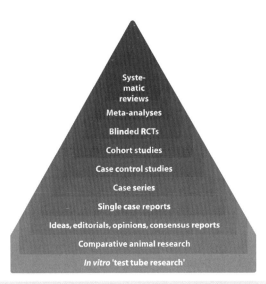

Fig. 2. Pyramid of evidence. This is a widely used representation of the quality of the evidence used to make clinical decisions. Items toward the top of the pyramid are considered to represent stronger sources of evidence, and those toward the base of the pyramid represent weaker sources of evidence.

observations. They do not compare the observations with a control group, and extreme caution should be practiced before using them to make conclusions about treatment effects. Their main use is to provide early reports of new phenomena and for formulating hypotheses that can be tested by more appropriate and powerful studies.

Readers should be aware that studies are occasionally published with misleading titles. It is not uncommon to find cohort studies with titles claiming them to be RCTs or case-control studies describing cohort studies or even case series. Clinical researchers may be forced to use a variation of one of the study designs described in this article for pragmatic reasons. A careful reading and appraisal of the methodology described in the paper should explain how and why the study was performed in this way and reveal the strengths and weaknesses of the study.

RESEARCH SYNTHESIS
Although the lack of a substantial base of primary research in small animal veterinary medicine makes it difficult to perform systematic reviews and meta-analyses, they nonetheless represent the strongest form of evidence in making clinical decisions.

Systematic Reviews
It is important to appreciate the difference between the traditional narrative review and a formally conducted systematic review. A narrative review represents

an author's subjective interpretation of the literature. It may represent a relatively balanced and objective survey of the literature, but there is no way for the reader to confirm this. The authors of a systematic review follow a strict protocol in the searching and appraisal of the literature to provide some guarantee of the thoroughness and objectivity of the review. They describe how the literature search was performed, and thus enable the reader to repeat that search to find more recent research data.

The work of the International/American College of Veterinary Dermatology Task Force on Canine Atopic Dermatitis has produced a series of systematic reviews, and the members of this task force are to be commended on their work. Their article entitled "Evidence-based veterinary dermatology: a systematic review of the pharmacotherapy of canine atopic dermatitis" [2] is a good example of this type of secondary research.

Meta-Analyses

A meta-analysis is a survey in which the designs of all the included studies are similar enough statistically that the results can be combined and analyzed as if they were a single study. When possible, a systematic review attempts to summarize the results of the papers reviewed in this manner. Sadly, it is rarely possible to find sufficient primary studies in the veterinary field that allow this to be done. For a meta-analysis to be performed, the studies must conform in the methodology used and in the populations being studied so as to make a formal statistical analysis meaningful.

An example of a meta-analysis performed examining the use of cyclosporine in the treatment of atopic dermatitis in dogs [3] provides a rare veterinary example of this type of systematic review.

The results of a meta-analysis are often presented in a forest plot indicating the odds ratio and the confidence intervals of the individual and combined studies. An example of a forest plot of a meta-analysis is shown in Fig. 3. An odds ratio of 1 indicates no effect. An odds ratio of greater than 1 indicates an improvement, and an odds ratio less than 1 indicates a worsening.

PRIMARY RESEARCH STUDIES

Randomized Controlled Trials

When choosing a therapy for a patient, the best evidence is likely to come from one or more RCTs. The overall design of a classic RCT is shown in Fig. 4.

The RCT has two important features. First, there are at least two groups, one or more treatment groups, and a control group. The treatment group receives the treatment or intervention under investigation, and the control group receives a placebo or a standard treatment. The second key feature of the RCT is that patients are randomly assigned to the two groups. The two groups are observed in an identical fashion. The groups are followed for a predetermined period, after which the trial ends. Double blinding should be used if possible. A trial in which neither the owner or animal nor the veterinary surgeon knows which treatment the animal is receiving is called a double-blind trial. This

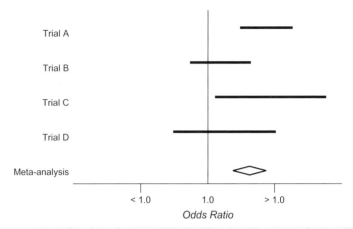

Fig. 3. Graphic representation of the results of a meta-analysis of four different clinical trials as a forest plot. The width of each bar indicates the confidence intervals of the result from each trial. The combined statistical analysis is shown as horizontal diamond shape, which also shows the confidence intervals of the overall result.

avoids bias and ensures that each group, whether treatment or control, has an equivalent placebo effect. The measured outcome therefore relates to the actual treatment rather than the act of merely providing a treatment.

The control group allows a comparison to be made between the treatment and a chosen alternative, such as no treatment or an existing accepted therapy. This is important, because an excellent cure rate without a control may simply reflect the outcome of the natural course of the disease irrespective of the treatment used.

Random allocation reduces the risk of bias; it is the most powerful method of eliminating known and unknown confounding variables, and increases the probability that the differences between the groups can be attributed to the treatment. It can be unethical to use an untreated control group if withholding an effective treatment leads to unnecessary suffering in these animals, however. RCTs are relatively expensive to conduct, and they require considerable labor and extensive planning if they are to be performed well.

Cross-Over Designs

Cross-over studies are a variation of the RCT and are useful for symptomatic treatments of more chronic conditions (Fig. 5). The subjects in the trial are randomly assigned to one of two treatment groups and followed over time to see if they develop the outcome of interest. After a period during which the outcome would have been expected to occur, they are switched to the other treatment. A washout period between the two treatments may be used to reduce the residual effects of the treatments or to establish the effect of no treatment. The subjects are then monitored for a further period, and the outcomes are noted.

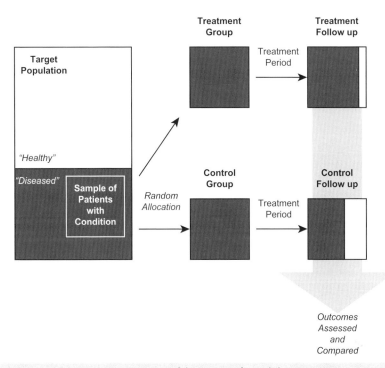

Fig. 4. Diagrammatic representation of the steps performed during an RCT.

Because the subjects act as their own controls, the number of animals required for the trial can be less than the number required for a standard RCT. Cross-over studies are not appropriate for all conditions and may be less useful for treatments with persistent actions.

Cohort Studies

Like the experimental studies described previously, observational studies (eg, cohort studies, case-control studies, cross-sectional surveys) are explanatory in nature, providing a comparison between two groups. Unlike experimental studies, however, the allocation of the subjects to the groups being compared is not under the control of the researcher. Allocation to the study groups is a result of the criteria decided on during the study design. For these reasons, the power of observational studies is reduced in comparison to experimental studies.

Observational studies allow studies to be performed that would be difficult to perform experimentally. For example, studies looking at the effect of weight in the incidence of kidney disease in cats would be expensive to study by experiment yet relatively inexpensive to investigate using observational designs. This type of study is often used to investigate risk factors in disease, for example, the development of urolithiasis and different types of feline diet.

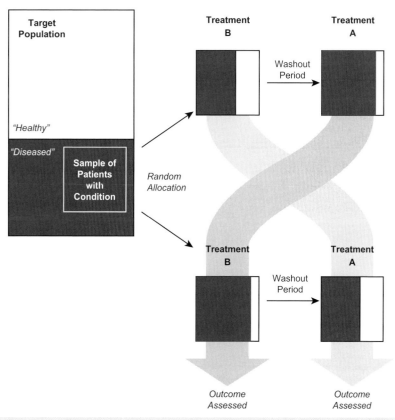

Fig. 5. Diagrammatic representation of the steps performed in the conduct of a cross-over study.

Cohort studies (Fig. 6) are those in which animals exposed to a putative causal factor are followed over time and compared with another group that is not exposed to that specific factor. The two groups are equally monitored for specific outcomes. A cohort study may also be used to compare outcomes from two different treatments (the RCT is the experimental equivalent of a cohort study). Both groups contain animals diagnosed with the disease under investigation, and the groups are defined by the treatment received. This type of study allows comparison of risk and intervention in a prospective manner when it is not possible to implement an RCT. For example, dogs with an amputated hind leg could be monitored for the development of osteoarthritis in the remaining hind leg over a 24-month period. These animals would be compared with a group of healthy dogs. The results should identify factors that are statistically overrepresented in either of the two cohorts.

Cohort studies are generally preferred to case-control studies because they are statistically more reliable. They are less expensive to perform than

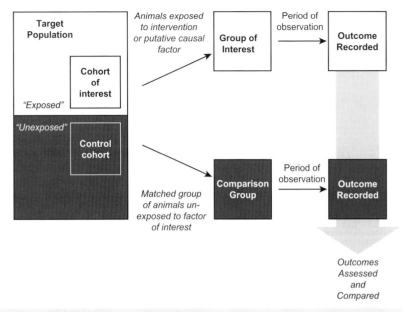

Fig. 6. Diagrammatic representation of the steps performed during a cohort study.

RCTs, and in comparison to case-control studies, they can provide evidence concerning the timing and sequence of events. When prospective cohort studies are performed, the data collection can be standardized, avoiding the incomplete data sets that may arise from the use of historical records.

Blinding is difficult to achieve in cohort studies, and an inability to "blind" may be the reason why a cohort design is selected. It may also be difficult to identify a matched control group to minimize other variables that may confound the results. Cohort studies are more prone to dropouts (when subjects are removed from the study because of subsequent death, removal by owners, or other events), and they are less useful for rare diseases, because it may be difficult to recruit a sufficiently large number of cases.

Case-Control Studies

As its name suggests, the two groups compared in a case-control study are "cases" and "controls." For the case group, animals that have developed a disease condition are identified and their exposure to suspected causal or risk factors is compared with that of a control group that does not have the disease (Fig. 7). Animals in the control group are matched with the cases to ensure that confounding factors that might influence the result are evenly distributed in the two groups. In a small animal study, factors like age, gender, breed, neutering, and vaccination status might be typically chosen in matching controls to cases. The matching may be performed as each case is identified, and an animal matching on age, breed, and gender, for example, may be chosen at random

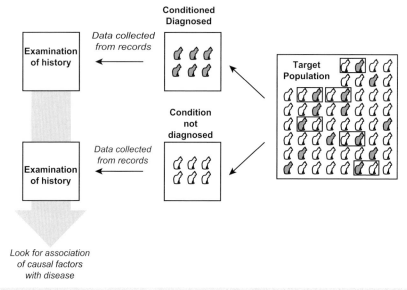

Fig. 7. Diagrammatic representation of the steps performed in the conduct of a case-control study.

from the clinical records of the hospital. Case-control studies are typically performed retrospectively using questionnaires or case records, and the information regarding exposure to risk factors is historical. For example, the diets of dogs with osteochondritis dissecans (OCD) could be compared with those of dogs that do not have OCD, and the owners could be asked to answer questions on the dietary and exercise histories of their animals. When a statistical relation between a risk factor and a condition is found, it does not necessarily mean that there is a causal relation. Case-control studies can also be used to provide evidence of whether an intervention has been effective or not. The results of case-control studies are normally expressed as odds ratios. Absolute risk from the overall population cannot be determined.

The main advantages of case-control studies are that they are quick to perform and do not require special methods to conduct. They are generally inexpensive and may be the only way in which rare conditions or those with a long incubation period can be realistically studied. Case-control studies are generally considered to be less reliable than RCTs or cohort studies, because it may be difficult to match the control group and eliminate confounding variables (because only known or suspected confounding variables can be controlled). It is not possible to calculate true incidence or prevalence and relative risk from case-control studies, but they are useful to formulate hypotheses that can be tested using further studies. Data in case-control studies are collected retrospectively, and records may be missing or of poor quality.

Cross-Sectional Surveys

In a cross-sectional survey, data can be used to determine a relation between exposure to a factor and the presence of disease. A representative sample of the whole population is chosen. Within the sample, two groups are identified, usually dividing the group into those animals with a specified disease and those without. Identical sets of parameters are then recorded for the two groups (Fig. 8). The strength of the relation between the disease and the parameter can then be expressed as an odds ratio. This is the only type of study that can yield true prevalence rates.

Cross-sectional surveys are relatively inexpensive to perform and present few ethical problems. No evidence of temporal relations can be obtained from these studies, however; thus, it is difficult to distinguish between cause and effect. Only association and lack of causation can be demonstrated, although when these associations are combined with our understanding of disease processes, they can produce quite strong circumstantial evidence for causation Cross-sectional surveys tend to generate hypotheses rather than to test hypotheses.

Diagnostic Tests and Screening Tests

Studies providing useful evidence for the selection of a diagnostic test may be derived from experimental or observational studies. The essential information

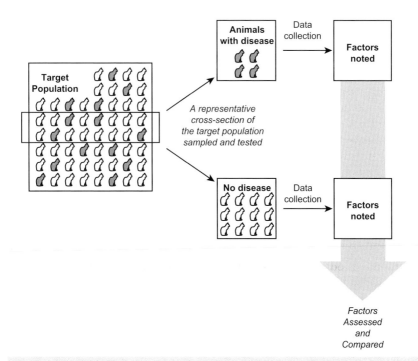

Fig. 8. Diagrammatic representation of the design of a cross-sectional survey.

needed from these studies is the test's sensitivity and specificity. The sensitivity is the frequency of a positive test result in the animals that have a specified disease. The specificity is the frequency of a negative test result in animals that do not have the disease. From this information, the likelihood ratio for the presence of the disease for a given result can be generated, as described in the article on statistics and evidence-based veterinary medicine by O'Connor and Evans elsewhere in this issue.

To determine the sensitivity of a test, a group of animals with the disease for which the test is being evaluated is required. Not only should they have the disease, but they should represent the various stages of the disease encountered in the population the test is intended for. To confirm that these animals have the disease a "gold (reference) standard" test is required that is "always right" (ie, has a specificity and sensitivity of 100%). This is almost impossible achieve (or to be sure of). Postmortem examinations may be the only effective gold standard for some studies. A second group, animals free from disease, is required is to determine the specificity. This group must not have the disease and, ideally, should represent the population on which the test is to be used (ie, contain the same proportions of healthy animals and the same levels of other diseases). Thus, although the sensitivity and specificity are independent of the prevalence of the disease(s) being tested, the groups should represent the population for which the test is going to be used. It is important that confidence intervals are determined for the results. The larger the number of animals in the groups, the narrower are the confidence intervals.

Poorly Controlled or Uncontrolled Trials

Occasionally, historical data from subjects that did not receive the treatment are used for comparison with a more recently treated experimental group. Historical controls often have poor outcomes and are rarely matched appropriately to the current treatment group. As a consequence, these comparisons often show the test treatment in a favorable light and should be viewed with caution, because there are many other variables that may have affected the result.

Studies that attempt to provide evidence for a treatment by comparing the outcomes from one hospital that uses one treatment with those of another hospital using an alternative treatment are of limited value. Although it is quite possible that there may be a genuine difference in outcomes from the treatments, it is not possible to eliminate other possibilities that might affect the treatment's efficacy and the magnitude of the difference can certainly not be relied on.

Most veterinarians have used the "treat and see" approach as a valid approach to establish the best therapy in the treatment of individual patients. Consider the treatment of osteoarthritis in the aging dog, in which there is a wide selection of treatment options. Although evidence is available in the literature, individual patient circumstances and variation in response sometimes mean that the best treatment is not always obvious. The veterinarian may commence treatment with a treatment for which there is good evidence of a desirable treatment outcome and be prepared to try several other treatments to establish the optimum therapy for the individual patient. To help make an objective decision, good patient records using well-defined descriptors should be used to record the outcomes of each treatment rather than relying on memory.

Trials may attempt to evaluate outcomes before and after an intervention has been introduced and assume that the difference between them is solely attributable to the intervention. This is a dangerous assumption, because there are many factors that are time dependent. The only type of study in which patients can be used reliably as their own controls is the cross-over study described previously.

Qualitative Research, Surveys, Case Reports, and Case Series

A full description of the advantages and disadvantages of qualitative research is beyond the scope of this short review. Surveys, case series, and case reports are different types of descriptive study that may be described as qualitative research. Most good clinical research is basic empiric research—studies in which measurements and counts are recorded as the result of observations and then subjected to statistical analysis. This type of research can be justly criticized on the basis that the investigator starts with a defined question. Good qualitative research can potentially reveal questions that would not otherwise have occurred to the investigator before embarking on the research. In some disciplines, such as ethology, sociology and psychology, qualitative research may be the best option in the investigation of complex systems. Fortunately, there remain many unanswered questions in veterinary clinical research that can easily be answered using quantitative research study designs.

Descriptive studies applied to populations of animals are called surveys. Properly conducted surveys are a form of cross-sectional study. Their objective is to provide data about the frequency of occurrence of a characteristic of interest, such as disease prevalence or the presence of a risk factor. It is important that the sample population is representative of the target population; in this regard, random sampling procedures are important to avoid bias.

A large proportion of the veterinary literature consists of case reports or case series (Fig. 9). A case report is a report on a single patient. A case series is a collection of case reports on the treatment of a condition or a clinical description of a condition.

A case report describes the presentation or course of a disease. It may be a novel presentation, an undocumented course of a familiar disease, or a description of a rare disease. The purpose of the report is to present a particular history, clinical description, diagnosis, treatment, or prognosis to the veterinary profession. A case series can provide descriptive quantitative data. They are useful in identifying the range and the frequencies of presentations that may be encountered. Descriptions of treatments and associated potential risk factors should be viewed with extreme caution and used to generate hypotheses only. Case series and case reports have no statistical validity, because there is no

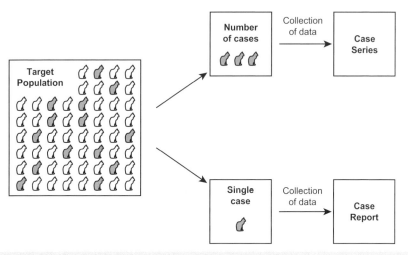

Fig. 9. Diagrammatic representation of case studies and case series.

control group, but they may be helpful if other sources of evidence are not available with regard to a rare condition. Case reports and case series are not usually regarded as research and are traditionally regarded as the lowest form of evidence. In the absence of other sources of information, however, they have an important role to play in the acquisition of evidence.

Case reports are convenient ways of describing rare complications of interventions that may not be documented in other research trials. Clearly, new and emerging diseases may be first described as a case report, and they may serve as early indicators of novel developments, risks, and diagnostic and therapeutic options. It is important to appreciate that the information provided has considerable limitations: the intervention described may not have influenced the outcome, there may be harm attached to the intervention, or the description may atypical of the rare disease. Readers should also realize that there may a publication bias in that promising or interesting interventions are published, whereas less striking or unpromising ones are not. The conclusions from these reports should be interpreted with considerable caution.

SUMMARY

It is probably appropriate to think again how we might consider ranking the evidence in the veterinary pyramid of evidence. There are occasions when all the evidence is contained in narrative reviews, book chapters, continuing education articles, and the like. There is no systematic method for comparing conflicting evidence from these sources, and veterinarians must use their own judgment on what constitutes the best evidence. When it comes to comparing the results of clinical research, we have to be pragmatic. Olivry and Mueller [2] categorized papers according to methodology and the number of subjects in each trial (Table 1). Their systematic review probably considered several papers that would be eliminated from a human medical systematic review because of methodologic flaws. Again, it falls to a veterinarian's own judgment how these flaws affect the evidence.

Further information about ranking evidence and the formal appraisal of evidence can be found in the article on critical appraisal of the evidence in scientific literature in this issue by Trevejo and elsewhere [4–7]. The key areas that all study designs should address are population, numbers, case definition, and bias.

Given the diverse nature of the species treated in small animal clinics, it is unlikely that the study population is going to be perfect for a decision involving one particular patient; however, the strength of evidence is improved if the population reflects those seen in your practice.

Case definition needs careful consideration. The qualities of diagnostic tests and diagnostic facilities available to veterinarians vary considerably. A well-designed clinical trial may be seriously flawed by a lack of attention to the precision or reliability of the diagnosis used.

The use of sufficient numbers of subjects in a trial is essential for the results to be statistically significant as described in the article on statistics and evidence-based veterinary medicine by Evans and O'Connor elsewhere in this issue. This is especially true of a negative result; the statistical power of the trial must be sufficient to have had a chance of detecting an effect had one existed.

The final area that good study designs are designed to eliminate is bias. Proper randomization rather than arbitrary choice is a good start. It takes little extra effort to create a random number list or to choose envelopes from a hat

Table 1
Categories used in the systematic review by Olivry and Mueller [2] to rank the relative strengths of different veterinary clinical research studies

Category	Study design	Subcategory
A	Blind randomized controlled trial (control with active drug or placebo)	(1) >50 subjects per group
		(2) 20–50 subjects per group
		(3) 10–19 subjects per group
		(4) <10 subjects per group
B	Controlled trial lacking blinding or randomization	(1) >50 subjects per group
		(2) 20–50 subjects per group
		(3) 10–19 subjects per group
		(4) <10 subjects per group
C	Open uncontrolled trial	(1) >50 subjects per group
		(2) 20–50 subjects per group
		(3) 10–19 subjects per group
		(4) <10 subjects per group
D	Cohort study, case-control analytic study, descriptive study, case report	(1) >50 subjects per group
		(2) 20–50 subjects per group
		(3) 10–19 subjects per group
		(4) <10 subjects per group

(or other convenient receptacle), and it is not the same as choosing every other patient to receive treatment A while giving treatment B to others. Careful consideration is required in selecting control groups and blinding, when at all possible, is an important factor in avoiding bias.

References

[1] American Academy of Pediatrics Task Force on Infant Positioning and SIDS. Positioning and SIDS: changing concepts of sudden infant death syndrome: implications for infant sleeping environment and sleep position. Pediatrics 1992;89:1120–6.

[2] Olivry T, Mueller RS. Evidence-based dermatology: a systematic review of the pharmacotherapy of canine atopic dermatitis. Vet Dermatol 2003;14:121–46.

[3] Steffan J, Favrot C, Mueller R. A systematic review and meta-analysis of the efficacy and safety of cyclosporin for the treatment of atopic dermatitis in dogs. Vet Dermatol 2006;17:3–16.

[4] Dahoo IR, Waltner-Toews D. Interpreting clinical research: part I. General considerations. Compendium of Continuing Education 1985;7(9):S474–7.

[5] Dahoo IR, Waltner-Toews D. 1985 Interpreting clinical research: part II. Descriptive and experimental studies. Compendium of Continuing Education 1985;7(9):S513–9.

[6] Dahoo IR, Waltner-Toews D. 1985 Interpreting clinical research: part III. Observational studies and interpretation of results. Compendium of Continuing Education 1985;7(9):S605–13.

[7] Cockroft PD, Holmes MA. Handbook of evidence-based veterinary medicine. Oxford (UK): Blackwells Scientific; 2003.

Vet Clin Small Anim 37 (2007) 463–475

VETERINARY CLINICS
SMALL ANIMAL PRACTICE

SEVIER
UNDERS

A Small Animal Clinician's Guide to Critical Appraisal of the Evidence in Scientific Literature

Rosalie T. Trevejo, DVM, MPVM, PhD

College of Veterinary Medicine, Western University of Health Sciences, 309 East 2nd Street, Pomona, CA 91766-1854, USA

As veterinary professionals, we access the scientific literature to keep abreast of medical advances and to assist us in making sound clinical decisions. When presented with data on topics such as new medical procedures, drug therapies, or vaccines, the clinician must evaluate the findings and determine if they offer a worthwhile advantage over any existing protocols. To evaluate the merits of reported findings, the reader must consider the type of study design used, determine the applicability of the findings to a particular patient or patient population, and take into account any other factors that may have influenced the study's conclusions.

The field of evidence-based medicine has helped to address the needs of veterinarians to appraise, synthesize, and use a myriad of scientific research [1,2]. The journal *Veterinary Dermatology* has adopted an evidence-based approach to its systematic review articles, using a predetermined rating system for the level of evidence, with randomized clinical trials considered to offer the strongest evidence [3]. This use of an established format to develop recommendations for the best approach to diagnose or treat a disease is an example of the use of evidence-based medicine as a decision-making tool.

The article on evaluation of evidence by Holmes in this issue presented the various types of study designs as a hierarchy of scientific evidence, with some studies carrying more scientific weight than others because of the inherent nature of their design. The current article illustrates the process of critically appraising the evidence presented in scientific reports, focusing on observational and experimental studies. The objectives of this article are to use real-life examples to familiarize the reader with (1) determining how well the study population represents the population of interest; (2) assessing the features of different study designs, including potential sources of bias; and (3) evaluating the statistical evidence.

E-mail address: rtrevejo@westernu.edu

0195-5616/07/$ – see front matter
doi:10.1016/j.cvsm.2007.01.005

STUDY POPULATION

When evaluating a scientific report, assuming the findings are correct for the population being studied, how do we determine the applicability of the findings to populations outside of the study population? In an ideal world, we would have data on the entire population of interest, removing any reservations we may have on making such inferences. Because the study population has been determined in large part by the investigator, however, it is important to consider how it was selected.

The generalizability of a study's findings to the source population from which the study participants were drawn is referred to as the external validity of the findings. The ultimate source of any study population is the general population. It is up to the investigator to identify the target population that has the characteristics of interest within the general population. The investigator then selects the study population from the target population. For example, if an investigator is planning a study of risk factors for pyometra in dogs, the general population would be the "universe" of the canine population and the target population would consist of female dogs. The investigator would then determine how to select the study population from the target population (ie, female dogs from randomly selected veterinary hospitals in the United States). The makeup of the study population depends on such factors as the amount of time and resources available to the investigator, accessibility of the target population, detectability of the condition of interest, and frequency of occurrence of the condition under study. Ideally, the study population should be selected in such as way as to maximize its generalizability to the target population.

A random sample is ideal for several reasons, with a major one being that it removes the chance of intentional or unintentional bias on the part of the investigator when selecting the study population. This approach requires a complete enumeration of the target population, which may not be available or may be too resource-intensive to assemble. For instance, to examine the association between enteric infections and feeding a raw meat diet to pet dogs in the United States, a random sample drawn from a list of all pet dogs in the United States would help to ensure representation of different geographic regions that may vary in their prevalence of enteric infections or feeding practices. When random sampling is not used, consideration must be given to how the methods used to select the study population may influence the study outcome. For instance, a study population may be selected from the proportion of the target population that was accessible to the investigator. In this case, a component of the target population may have been eligible for inclusion in the study but was not available to or sought out by the investigator.

Many studies use a convenience sample, such as a patient population seen at a particular facility, such as a teaching hospital. This results in a study population that may differ from that of the target population. For instance, study participants from a teaching hospital likely overrepresent severe or complicated cases of the disease or condition under study, with resultant underrepresentation of milder or subclinical cases. The extreme example is the case report or case series, which can add to our existing knowledge by reporting on a new or unusual disease presentation. A case report or case series typically contains information from cases that were observed by the investigator and are unlikely to be representative of all cases of that particular disease or condition in the general population. Nevertheless, they are useful for generating hypotheses about potential risk factors for the observed condition and for stimulating future studies to describe the extent of disease occurrence (descriptive studies) or to assess potential risk factors or interventions (analytic studies) quantitatively in the population of interest.

STUDY DESIGN CONSIDERATIONS

There are two major categories of study designs: observational (cross-sectional, case-control, and cohort studies) and experimental (randomized control trial). A major difference between these categories is the amount of control exerted by the investigator. In the former, disease and exposure status are observed and described, whereas in the latter, they can be assigned by the investigator. Each type of study design has potential limitations that can be minimized through careful planning by the investigator. Important questions to ask of any type of study are how the outcome (ie, disease) is defined, whether the outcome is readily measurable, and, if applicable, whether an appropriate control group was used. An important consideration for the investigator when selecting a study design is the level of existing knowledge. For instance, when relatively little is known about a disease, a descriptive study, such as a cross-sectional study, may be indicated to gather basic information, such as the prevalence of a condition in the population, and to detect patterns, such as breed or age distribution.

As an example, West Nile virus (WNV) was first detected in the Western Hemisphere after a 1999 outbreak in New York that resulted in morbidity and mortality among human beings, horses, and birds. Kile and colleagues [4] used a cross-sectional study design to conduct a serosurvey of dogs and cats during a 2002 outbreak of WNV in Louisiana and to identify environmental factors associated with seropositivity to WNV. A convenience sample was taken of dogs and cats evaluated at veterinary facilities (family owned) or animal shelters (strays). Serum samples from 116 (26%) of 442 dogs and 13 (9%) of 138 cats yielded positive results. Outdoor-only family dogs were almost 19 times as likely to be seropositive for WNV compared with indoor-only family dogs, and stray dogs were almost twice as likely to be seropositive compared with family dogs. Family dogs receiving heartworm medication were less likely to be seropositive for WNV compared with family dogs not receiving heartworm medication.

This study yielded descriptive data on a newly emerging disease in the Western Hemisphere and explored possible environmental risk factors for seropositivity. Because the dogs and cats in this serosurvey were a convenience sample rather than a representation of the pet population in the outbreak area, it is not possible to generalize the findings to all pet dogs and cats in the area.

Nevertheless, a large difference in seropositivity between dogs and cats was demonstrated. The authors hypothesize that the lower seropositivity rates in cats compared with dogs may result from mosquito feeding preferences and cats being less tolerant of feeding mosquitoes than dogs. Another finding was the apparent protective effect of heartworm medication, which was also raised as an issue that warrants further examination. These findings demonstrate the utility of a descriptive study design to gain a better understanding of a disease and to generate additional hypotheses for study that deserve further investigation.

Experimental Study Design

Experimental studies, such as the randomized clinical trial, are considered to be at the top of the hierarchy of study designs for several reasons. For one, because the treatments are administered under controlled conditions and the outcome is measured prospectively, there is a strong basis for establishment of cause and effect. The investigator should be blinded to the treatment status of study participants to prevent this knowledge from systematically influencing the evaluation of study outcomes, a form of study bias. Bias may also occur during randomized control trials when the selection criteria for including patients in a study do not ensure uniformity of individuals (selection bias), when patients that leave a study differ systematically from those that remain (migration bias), or when uniform standards for measuring study outcomes cannot be maintained over time (measurement bias) [5]. The randomization of study participants to treatment groups allows for control of known and unknown influences, such as differences in severity of illness between the treatment and control groups. It may not always be ethical to randomize, however, particularly if some patients are randomized to a group receiving no treatment for a disease. Instead, patients can be randomly assigned to receive different treatments for comparison.

As an example, analgesics are indicated in patients undergoing painful procedures, such as cats undergoing onychectomy. Romans and colleagues [6] randomized 27 client- or shelter-owned cats to receive one of three postoperative analgesic protocols after unilateral onychectomy of the left forelimb: topical bupivacaine, intramuscular administration of butorphanol, or transdermal administration of fentanyl. The outcome was gait analysis, with force as a percentage of body weight measured on a pressure platform (Fig. 1). The results indicate that cats treated with butorphanol or fentanyl had significantly better limb function after onychectomy compared with cats treated with topical bupivacaine.

This study provides an example in which inclusion of a control group that did not receive any analgesia would not be considered ethical because of the painful nature of the procedure. The inclusion of client- and shelter-owned cats in the study raises the possibility of selection bias if these two populations differ with respect to reaction to stress or pain and they were differentially assigned to the different treatment groups. The investigators do not indicate whether the person conducting the gait analysis was blinded to the treatment

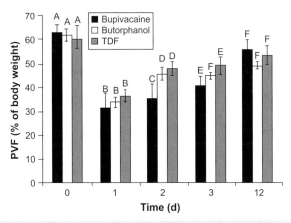

Fig. 1. Mean peak vertical force (PVF) of the left forelimb, expressed as a percentage of body weight, in cats that underwent unilateral onychectomy and received bupivacaine topically (n = 9), butorphanol intramuscularly (n = 9), or fentanyl transdermally (TDF; n = 8) for postoperative analgesia. Error bars represent the standard error of the mean. Columns with different letters were significantly (P<.05) different. (*From* Romans CW, Gordon WJ, Robinson DA, et al. Effect of postoperative analgesic protocol on limb function following onychectomy in cats. J Am Vet Med Assoc 2005;227:90; with permission.)

status of each patient. The likelihood of measurement bias in this study was reduced by the use of gait analysis to evaluate study outcomes, however, because the pressure platform would provide a result that is objective and readily measurable. The following example of another randomized clinical trial to evaluate postoperative analgesia after onychectomy in cats illustrates the potential for measurement bias.

Curcio and colleagues [7] conducted a study of postoperative analgesia protocols after bilateral onychectomy, in which experienced observers, who were blinded to the treatment status, assigned a discomfort score based on observed lameness, foot reaction, and pain. In this study, 20 cats were given intramuscular buprenorphine before surgery. In addition, one forelimb of each cat was randomized to receive bupivacaine as a four-point regional nerve block. An advantage of assigning different treatments to different forelimbs of the same cat is the ability to control for variation between cats in response to the same analgesic protocol. Because both forelimbs would be expected to be painful, however, this design may minimize the ability to detect a difference between the two protocols. No difference in discomfort score was detected between the control and treatment limbs in this study. The outcome measure (discomfort score) could be subjective and depend on which observer was taking the measurement, however (Table 1). Bias would be a concern in this study if the observers had not been blinded to the postoperative analgesia assignment of each forelimb. The observers were blinded in this study, however, which minimized the possibility of bias in assessing the outcome.

Table 1
Scoring system used for assessment of signs of discomfort after forelimb onychectomy in cats (n = 20) after receiving buprenorphine (0.01 mg/kg [0.004 mg/lb] administered intramuscularly), in which one forelimb received bupivacaine (1 mg/kg [0.45 mg/lb] of a 0.75% solution) administered as a four-point regional nerve block and the other forelimb was used as a control

Variable	Score
Foot reaction	0 = Not bothering feet
	1 = Shaking feet
	2 = Licking feet
	3 = Chewing feet
Lameness	0 = None
	1 = Mild
	2 = Marked
	3 = Touching toe
	4 = Not weight bearing
Signs of pain	0 = None
	1 = Resists firm touching
	2 = Resists moderate touching
	3 = Resists mild touching
	4 = Severe, resists any touching

Data from Curcio K, Bidwell LA, Bohart GV, et al. Evaluation of signs of postoperative pain and complications after forelimb onychectomy in cats receiving buprenorphine alone or with bupivacaine administered as a four-point regional nerve block. J Am Vet Med Assoc 2006;228:65–8.

Observational Study Design

In general, observational studies are less expensive and more practical to conduct than experimental studies, and thus tend to be the most widely used. As discussed in the previous article by Holmes, the major types of observational studies include cross-sectional, case-control, and cohort studies. The resources available to the investigator (ie, time, money), the frequency of the disease, and the level of preexisting knowledge about the disease can all determine what type of observational study is best suited for the disease or condition under study. Systematic errors (bias) that result in an incorrect estimate of the association between exposure and risk of disease can occur with each of the observational study designs [8]. The two general types of bias result from (1) using inconsistent criteria to enroll participants in a study and (2) obtaining noncomparable information from the different study groups. The specific types of bias that can occur with the different types of study designs are discussed in more detail for each respective study type.

Cross-sectional study

In the cross-sectional study design, the study population is assessed at a point in time with respect to disease and exposure to various potential risk factors. It offers a convenient and relatively inexpensive method for measuring disease prevalence and detecting potential risk factors for disease, as illustrated by the previous example of the WNV serosurvey [4]. Because exposure status and disease are ascertained simultaneously, a limitation of this study design is the lack of evidence that a putative risk factor actually caused the disease. In addition, the duration of the disease or condition under study influences the measure of disease prevalence, such that diseases of long duration are more likely to be detected than those of short duration. Information bias is a potential problem in cross-sectional studies if the investigator's knowledge of the participant's disease or exposure status at the time of data collection results in systematic differences in the soliciting, recording, or interpreting of information from the study participant [8]. Another potential type of bias results from misclassification, which occurs if participants are erroneously categorized with respect to disease or exposure status. When the misclassification depends on the disease or exposure status, over- or underestimation of the association between disease and exposure can result.

As an example, feline leukemia virus (FeLV) and feline immunodeficiency virus (FIV) are among the most common infectious diseases of cats in North American. Levy and colleagues [9] conducted a cross-sectional study to determine the seroprevalence of FeLV and FIV infection among cats in North America and risk factors for seropositivity. Potential study centers in the United States and Canada were identified through the membership roster of the American Association of Feline Practitioners; a list of all individuals who had recently purchased FeLV and FIV test kits; and lists of animal shelters, cat rescue organizations, and groups participating in trap-neuter-return programs for feral cats derived from various Internet directories. From August through November 2004, participating study centers (345 veterinary clinics and 145 animal shelters) submitted results of FeLV and FIV testing performed on 18,038 cats and kittens, of which 2.3% were seropositive for FeLV and 2.5% were seropositive for FIV. A multivariable analysis indicated that seropositivity was associated with age (adults more likely than juveniles), gender (sexually intact male cats more likely than sexually intact female cats), and health status (outdoor cats sick at the time of testing more likely than healthy indoor cats).

The investigators recruited study centers to represent major segments of the population that would be expected to test cats for FeLV and FIV. The report did not include data on the number of study sites the investigators attempted to recruit and the proportion successfully recruited from each of the subgroups of interest, such as geographic region and facility type, which are necessary for assessing the representativeness of the study population. Bias could result if exposure or disease is distributed differently between participating and nonparticipating centers. The investigators note that generalizability of the findings is limited, because the cats and study centers were not selected in a random manner. The use of the number of cats tested as the denominator for calculation of rates may have biased the results toward cats at higher risk if cats that were presented to the study centers but were not tested had a lower risk of infection. Similarly, if veterinarians were more likely to promote testing for high-risk cats that were presented to their clinics, the study results for these cats may be biased toward cats at a higher risk. Alternatively, the investigators note that shelters may have been more likely to test healthy cats if they were perceived to be good candidates for adoption, resulting in an underestimation of the seroprevalence in this segment of the feline population.

Case-control studies

Case-control studies are an efficient design to compare the frequency of potential risk factors between diseased (case) and nondiseased (control) groups. They are ideal for the study of rare diseases or those with a long latency period, because the investigator can actively identify cases rather than waiting for them to occur. In addition, case-control studies allow for the study of multiple potential risk factors. Case-control studies are susceptible to bias if cases and controls do not have an equal likelihood of being detected as cases if they develop the condition of interest (selection bias) or if there is better recollection of exposure for those cases with the disease (recall bias), which is a concern if client interviews are used to collect exposure information [10].

As an example, cranial cruciate ligament (CCL) injury is recognized as a common cause of hind limb lameness in dogs. In a case-control study to identify risk factors for rupture of the CCL among dogs younger than 2 years of age, Duval and colleagues [11] reviewed medical records from the teaching hospitals at the University of Georgia, Michigan State University, and the University of Pennsylvania to identify cases and age-matched controls. Dogs with rupture of the CCL were significantly more likely to be large breeds, such as the Neapolitan Mastiff, Akita, Saint Bernard, Rottweiler, Mastiff, Newfoundland, Chesapeake Bay Retriever, Labrador Retriever, and American Staffordshire Terrier, compared with the control group (Table 2). In addition, dogs

Table 2
Odds ratios and 95% confidence intervals for breeds of dogs represented by two or more cases of rupture of the CCL at less than 2 years old

Breed	No. case dogs	No. control Dogs	Odds ratio	95% confidence interval
Neapolitan Mastiff	3	0	15.33	1.68–139.85
Akita	6	2	11.69	3.32–41.13
Saint Bernard	5	2	9.84	2.52–38.41
Rottweiler	36	24	6.92	4.26–11.24
Mastiff	5	3	6.72	1.89–23.86
Newfoundland	10	6	6.65	2.74–16.12
Chesapeake Bay Retriever	4	3	5.11	1.33–19.69
Labrador Retriever	57	56	5.05	3.45–7.41
American Staffordshire Terrier	6	7	3.46	1.23–9.79
Chow Chow	4	6	2.51	0.75–9.03
English Bulldog	6	6	2.15	0.8–5.76

Data from Duval JM, Budsberg SC, Flo GL, et al. Breed, sex, and body weight as risk factors for rupture of the cranial cruciate ligament in young dogs. J Am Vet Med Assoc 1999;215:811–4.

with rupture of the CCL had significantly greater body weights than control dogs.

The selected control group used by Duval and colleagues [11] provides a good comparison, because the controls were presented at the same facility for presumably unrelated conditions, making it more likely that these two groups represent the same populations. The breed-specific odds ratios used to identify high-risk breeds are calculated using small numbers for many of the breeds, however, which produces estimates that are less precise (wider confidence intervals). One method of addressing this would be to combine breeds that occur in small numbers into larger groups with similar characteristics for purposes of comparison rather than attempting to examine each breed separately. This study also illustrates the limitation of the case-control study design for distinguishing whether a putative risk factor actually caused the disease. For instance, the investigators conclude that greater body weight may have predisposed dogs to rupture of the CCL. The median duration of clinical signs before evaluation was 4.7 months, however, so it is possible that the association between rupture of the CCL and increased weight may have resulted, at least in part, from weight gain attributable to inactivity after the injury.

Cohort studies

In a cohort study, the study participants are classified by exposure status at the study onset and followed to compare the rate of disease occurrence in the exposure groups. Because exposure status is ascertained before the onset of disease, the cohort study provides stronger evidence of causality. A cohort study is not an ideal study design for rare diseases, however, because a prohibitive number of study participants may be required to ensure adequate numbers of cases. In addition, this study design is not amendable to the study of multiple potential risk factors because this could require the establishment of a prohibitive number of exposure subgroups. A major source of bias in cohort studies is loss to follow-up if those lost to follow-up differ from those that remain in the study with respect to disease or exposure [8].

Retrospective cohort studies are an option in cases in which good patient records exist, with documentation of the time of disease onset and exposure to risk factors under study. A potential source of bias in retrospective cohort studies occurs when the investigator is more or less likely to record the outcome of interest for participants with the exposure under study (interviewer bias) [8]. Selection bias, in which the selection of exposed or unexposed participants is related to their development of the outcome of interest, is a particular concern with retrospective cohort studies, because exposure and outcome are known at the outset of the study.

As an example, prepuberal gonadectomy is one approach to addressing the overpopulation problem in dogs and cats, although many veterinarians have concerns about outcomes, such as behavioral problems, urinary incontinence in female dogs, and obesity. Howe and colleagues [12] used a cohort study design to compare the long-term results of gonadectomy, in which dogs from two humane societies were classified into exposure groups based on the animal's age at the time of surgery: prepubertal (<24 weeks old) or traditional (≥24 weeks old) age. Dogs that were subsequently adopted out were eligible for inclusion in the study. Adoption records for dogs were used to follow up with owners at approximately 48 months after adoption. No difference was found in the incidence of physical or behavioral problems between the two age groups.

The process of interviewing owners by telephone to assess outcomes (physical or behavioral problems) in the dogs is likely to be less reliable than direct examination or medical record reviews. To improve the accuracy of the follow-up data, the investigators followed up with the treating veterinarian when the owner reported complex medical problems. It is possible that less serious or untreated conditions that may be related to the exposure were undetected by the investigators, however. Fifty eight percent of adopted dogs were lost to follow-up, raising the possibility that dogs lost to follow-up may have differed from those included in the study. No comparison was provided of the distribution of such factors as age, breed, or gender for the study participants versus those lost to follow-up, which would be useful for assessing whether there are major differences between these two groups. It is possible that selection bias may have played a role if the humane agencies selectively referred traditional age dogs for surgery if they were perceived to be more adoptable (ie, no behavioral problems, good physical health). If prepubertal gonadectomy does indeed increase the risk of behavioral or physical problems, the selection of traditional age dogs that were less likely to have these problems would have maximized the observed differences between the groups. Nevertheless, because no significant difference was found between the two exposure groups, the presence of this particular bias would provide further support of the observed findings.

EVALUATING THE STATISTICAL EVIDENCE

Because it is rarely possible for an investigator to include every member of a population in a study, a target population is typically sampled to create the study population. Assuming that the study population was selected in a way to minimize bias, the investigators can use the findings to make an inference about the target population. The accuracy of the inference is largely determined by the sample size, in which a larger sample size increases the reliability of the inference and decreases the variability in the estimate. When a study indicates that there is an association between an exposure and a disease (ie, odds ratio >1), there is always a possibility that this finding is attributable to chance. There are two components to evaluating the role of chance: (1) performing a test of statistical significance to determine the likelihood that sampling variability played a role in the observed results and (2) calculating the confidence interval, which indicates the range within which the true estimate of effect is likely to lie with a given degree of assurance (usually 95%) [13].

The study question must be framed as a hypothesis before conducting a test of statistical significance. This consists of a null hypothesis, which states that there is no association between an exposure and a disease, and an alternate hypothesis, which states that there is an association. The type of statistical test used depends on the particular situation [14]. The article by Evans and O'Connor on statistics and evidence-based medicine in this issue addresses specific types of statistical tests in detail. The sample size and the difference between the observed study values and those expected under the null hypothesis factor into the calculation of any test statistic [13].

Statistical testing yields a probability statement (*P* value) that indicates the probability of obtaining a result at least as extreme as the observed result by chance alone, assuming that the null hypothesis is true. A statistically significant *P* value is typically set by the investigator at .05 or less, indicating that there is at most a 5% probability of observing an association at least as extreme by chance alone, assuming that the null hypothesis is true. The investigator can select whatever *P* value cutoff is most appropriate, however, depending on how conservative he or she wishes to be. When statistical testing yields a small *P* value ($\leq$.05), this indicates that chance is less likely to have played a role in the findings and the null hypothesis is rejected in favor of the alternative hypothesis that an association exists. The actual *P* value should always be reported, because a *P* value that is only slightly higher than the conventional level of *P* = .05 (ie, *P* = .07) would be reported as nonsignificant but is close to statistical significance and may have been with a larger sample size [13]. For example, a case-control study to examine the effect of dietary vegetable consumption on reducing the risk of transitional cell carcinoma of the urinary bladder in Scottish Terriers found that consumption of cruciferous vegetable three or more times per week was associated with a 78% reduction in risk (odds ratio = 0.22; *P* = .07) [15]. Although this association was not considered statistically significant, it was based on a small sample size with two cases and eight controls reported as having the exposure of interest, indicating the need for further study with a larger sample size.

The confidence interval represents the range within which the true magnitude of effect lies with a specified degree of assurance. It is useful for evaluating the role of chance while also providing a measure of the amount of variability of the estimate attributable to the sample size. Ideally, the investigator should provide the confidence interval in conjunction with the *P* value. When interpreting the confidence interval, the first thing to determine is whether it contains the null value (ie, odds ratio = 1), indicating no association. When statistical significance is set at *P*$\leq$.05, a confidence interval containing the null value corresponds to *P*>.05. Second, the width of the confidence interval is inversely proportional to the sample size and reflects the amount of variability in the estimate. A narrow confidence interval that contains the null value is strong evidence that there is no association between the exposure and disease, whereas the role of chance is more difficult to rule out with a wide confidence interval [13].

In addition to considering the role of chance when evaluating the results of statistical testing, the reader must consider whether the statistical significance of an association between an exposure and a disease has biologic plausibility. For instance, an extremely small difference that is not clinically relevant may seem statistically significant if a large enough sample size is used. Another consideration is the use of multiple tests of statistical significance to evaluate the role of multiple potential risk factors [13]. The likelihood of finding a statistically significant result by chance alone is increased as the number of variables tested is increased. For example, Ward and colleagues [16] conducted a case-control study to evaluate environmental risk factors for leptospirosis in dogs. They evaluated 15 potential environmental risk factors, such as the presence of streams, wetlands, or flooding. Three of the 15 potential risk factors were significantly associated with a diagnosis of leptospirosis, whereas restriction of cases to those with a specific serovar (grippotyphosa) increased the number of significant risk factors to 7.

As discussed previously, the sample size is a major determinant of the magnitude of the role of chance when studying the potential association between an exposure and disease. When planning a study, the investigators must determine the number of study subjects necessary to ensure a given probability of detecting a statistically significant effect of a given magnitude if one truly exists [13]. Conversely, if the investigator is limited to a set number of study participants, a related question is how likely a statistically significant effect of a given magnitude is to be identified if present. When calculating sample sizes, the acceptable level of error must be selected a priori. The two types of errors are type I (α), which is the probability of rejecting the null hypothesis when it is true, and type II (β), which is the probability of failing to reject the null hypothesis when it is false. The probability of making a type I error is equal to the P value. Both types of error should ideally be minimized in a study. The power of a study is the probability of rejecting the null hypothesis when there is a true association between the disease and exposure and is equal to 1 minus β. The sample size is proportional to the level of power for a given study. There are many resources available to assist with sample size and power calculations [17–19].

SUMMARY

Although the evidence from randomized clinical trials is considered to be at the top of the hierarchy of evidence, they are not always feasible, ethical, or cost-effective to conduct. Observational studies, such as cross-sectional, case-control, and cohort studies, can also be valuable sources of information. Using the principles discussed in the current article can assist the reader in assessing the limitations of randomized clinical trials and observational studies. Evidence-based medicine and critical appraisal are recognized as important tools in the medical field, with many medical journals endorsing this approach for systematic review articles [3,20]. Through familiarity with the concepts of the selection of study populations, features of the different study designs, potential sources of study bias, and evaluation of the statistical evidence, the reader is well armed to start critically appraising the medical literature.

References

[1] Olivry T, Mueller RS. Evidence-based veterinary dermatology: a systematic review of the pharmacotherapy of canine atopic dermatitis. Vet Dermatol 2003;14(3):121–46.

[2] Evidence Based Medicine Toolkit. Internet citation [April 11, 2003]; Available at: http://www.med.ualberta.ca/ebm/ebm.htm. Accessed June 29, 2006.

[3] Moriello KA. Editor's commentary: introducing evidence based clinical reviews in veterinary dermatology. Vet Dermatol 2003;14(3):119–20.

[4] Kile JC, Panella NA, Komar N, et al. Serologic survey of cats and dogs during an epidemic of West Nile virus infection in humans. J Am Vet Med Assoc 2005;226(8):1349–53.

[5] Smith RD. Design and evaluation of clinical trials. In: Veterinary clinical epidemiology. 3rd edition. Boca Raton (FL): CRC Press; 2006. p. 127–35.

[6] Romans CW, Gordon WJ, Robinson DA, et al. Effect of postoperative analgesic protocol on limb function following onychectomy in cats. J Am Vet Med Assoc 2005;227(1):89–93.

[7] Curcio K, Bidwell LA, Bohart GV, et al. Evaluation of signs of postoperative pain and complications after forelimb onychectomy in cats receiving buprenorphine alone or with bupivacaine administered as a four-point regional nerve block. J Am Vet Med Assoc 2006;228(1): 65–8.

[8] Hennekens CH, Buring JE. Analysis of epidemiologic studies: evaluating the role of bias. In: Mayrent SL, editor. Epidemiology in medicine. 1st edition. Boston: Little, Brown and Company; 1987. p. 272–86.

[9] Levy JK, Scott HM, Lachtara JL, et al. Seroprevalence of feline leukemia virus and feline immunodeficiency virus infection among cats in North America and risk factors for seropositivity. J Am Vet Med Assoc 2006;228(3):371–6.

[10] Smith RD. Risk assessment and prevention. In: Veterinary clinical epidemiology. Boca Raton (FL): CRC Press; 2006. p. 91–109.

[11] Duval JM, Budsberg SC, Flo GL, et al. Breed, sex, and body weight as risk factors for rupture of the cranial cruciate ligament in young dogs. J Am Vet Med Assoc 1999;215(6):811–4.

[12] Howe LM, Slater MR, Boothe HW, et al. Long-term outcome of gonadectomy performed at an early age or traditional age in dogs. J Am Vet Med Assoc 2001;218(2):217–21.

[13] Hennekens CH. Evaluating the role of chance. In: Mayrent SL, editor. Epidemiology in medicine. 1st edition. Boston: Little, Brown and Company; 1987. p. 243–86.

[14] Smith RD. Statistical significance. In: Veterinary clinical epidemiology. 3rd edition. Boca Raton (FL): CRC Press; 2006. p. 127–61.

[15] Raghavan M, Knapp DW, Bonney PL, et al. Evaluation of the effect of dietary vegetable consumption on reducing risk of transitional cell carcinoma of the urinary bladder in Scottish Terriers. J Am Vet Med Assoc 2005;227(1):94–100.

[16] Ward MP, Guptill LF, Wu CC. Evaluation of environmental risk factors for leptospirosis in dogs: 36 cases (1997–2002). J Am Vet Med Assoc 2004;225(1):72–7.

[17] Sample size calculations to plan an experiment. Available at: http://www.graphpad.com/index.cfm?cmd=library.page&pageID=19&categoryID=4. Accessed June 30, 2006.

[18] Simon S. Quick sample size calculations. Available at: http://www.childrens-mercy.org/stats/size/quick.asp. Accessed June 30, 2006.

[19] Sample Size Calculator. The survey system. Available at: http://www.surveysystem.com/sscalc.htm. Accessed June 30, 2006.

[20] Cook DJ, Mulrow CD, Haynes RB. Systematic reviews: synthesis of best evidence for clinical decisions. Ann Intern Med 1997;126(5):376–80.

Vet Clin Small Anim 37 (2007) 477–486

VETERINARY CLINICS
SMALL ANIMAL PRACTICE

Statistics and Evidence-Based Veterinary Medicine: Answers to 21 Common Statistical Questions That Arise from Reading Scientific Manuscripts

Richard B. Evans, PhD*, Annette O'Connor, BVSc, MVSc, Dvsc

Veterinary Diagnostic and Production Animal Medicine, Iowa State University College of Veterinary Medicine, Ames, IA 50011, USA

> A distinctive function of statistics is this: it enables the scientist to make a numerical evaluation of the uncertainty of his conclusion.
> —George Snedecor
> In theory there is no difference between theory and practice. In practice there is.
> —Yogi Berra

Evidence-based veterinary medicine relies critically on the scientific validity of research. A component of validity is the statistical design and subsequent analysis of data collected during the study. Correct statistical design reduces bias and improves generalizability, and correct analysis leads to appropriate inferences. Inference is the art and science of making correct decisions based on data. Because veterinarians are responsible for the medical care of their patents, it is also their responsibility to understand inferences about treatments presented in papers.

It is generally difficult to know if a statistical test is really the correct one for data presented in a paper. This is because space restrictions on scientific papers preclude detailed descriptions of the data and verification of test or model assumptions.

Wrong inferences can sometimes be identified, because the structure of the data is inconsistent with the test or the wrong conclusions are drawn from a statistical test. Common errors include treating correlated data as independent, treating discrete data as continuous, and misinterpreting what a statistical test is actually testing.

Research papers of general interest to clinical veterinarians are ones that investigate the effects of treatments on groups of subjects. When you read a

*Corresponding author. E-mail address: revans@iastate.edu (R.B. Evans).

0195-5616/07/$ – see front matter
doi:10.1016/j.cvsm.2007.01.006

paper, the first question to ask is how the groups are different. Most researchers and readers assume that a statistical test is comparing group means, but statistical tests can compare many different statistics and there are many parameters that could be different among groups. If the data are skewed, the median may be the parameter of interest, and it may sometimes be important to know if the variation is different among groups. Also, the groups may or may not be statistically significant but may be clinically significant. Although clinical significance is often subjective, some have made an attempt to make it more objective [1].

This article is designed to assist veterinarians with the interpretation and understanding of statistics presented in papers.

QUESTIONS

1. What is the difference between a sample average and a population mean?
   The population mean is a fixed but unknown quantity that is estimated by the sample average. Interest is in the population mean rather than in the sample average because it represents the central value for all subjects. The sample average is the average of the data for a particular sample and would change for a different sample. When two treatment groups are being compared, the sample averages of the groups are almost always different even though the population means of the two groups could be the same. That is because sampling variability influences the data.

2. What is a P value?
   A P value is a number between 0 and 1 that is used to quantify the authenticity of a statistical study hypothesis. Experiments or clinical studies use samples from populations of subjects to evaluate study group differences. Although the sample may be representative of the larger population, large variability in the population may weaken inferences obtained from samples. In other words, one cannot be sure if the differences seen among study groups are attributable to the experimental effects or to the variability naturally seen in the population. P values measure the strength of the inference. A small P value (traditionally less than .05) indicates that the result is real and not illusory [1]. Large P values indicate that the study result may have occurred because of the sampling variability rather than the effect of different study groups.
   When a P value is less than a set value (usually .05 but sometimes .1 or .01), it is called statistically significant, which means that the researcher believes the results of the study are real. That does not mean that study results have an impact on animal health in a meaningful way, however. Although the study result may be real, it may not have a large clinical effect, that is, not be clinically useful. Jacobsen and Truax [1] have investigated quantitative ways of defining clinical significance, and the concept is to compare the effect of treatment relative to the distributions of the diseased and nondiseased populations.

3. Why is a P value less than .05 considered statistically significant?
   Most veterinary research articles use .05 as a cutoff for "statistical significance" (see question 2). R.A. Fisher wrote, "We shall not often be astray

if we draw a conventional line at 0.05" [2]. P values are a continuum between 0 and 1 representing the strength of the statistical hypothesis. The cutoff of .05 is arbitrary, and there is not much difference in probability between .045 and .055. As a reader of researcher papers, it is important to realize that P values that are close to each other represent essentially the same evidentiary value. Drawing a firm line at an arbitrary cutoff may discard some promising therapies unnecessarily.

4. What is a t test?

T tests, also called the Student's t-test (named after the pen name of the person who developed the test), are used when there are two groups of independent study subjects and the data are continuous (eg, body weight) rather than discrete (eg, lameness score).

The objective of using a t test is to compare the means of two populations of subjects. It is never possible to measure every subject in a population, for example, to weigh all Labrador Retrievers; thus, populations are sampled to provide fewer but representative members, and the t test is used to infer the results from the sample of the study to the entire population. Typically, the population is sampled and divided into two treatment groups. For example, 40 hunting Labrador Retrievers may be sampled from regional kennel clubs and divided into two groups, with one group receiving a nutritional supplement and the other a placebo. The outcome variable may be the change in weight after several months during hunting season.

A t test returns a P value (see questions 2 and 3); if the P value is small, there is a difference among the group means that is greater than that attributable to chance.

Sometimes researchers use t tests for scale data (eg, body condition score). The old rule of thumb is that if the scale data have five levels, t tests can be used to compare the equality of the means of independent groups. This works when the sample size is reasonably large and the outcomes are distributed over the range of the scale.

A better test for two groups of scale data is the χ^2 test [3]. It does not compare group means, however, but rather the distribution of scale values between the groups; therefore, the interpretation of a small P value resulting from a χ^2 test would be different. If could even be the case that the sample averages of two groups of scale data are the same but that the χ^2 tests reports a P value less than .05, indicating group differences.

5. What is ANOVA?

ANOVA is the acronym for analysis of variance, which is a method of comparing population means of independent groups of independent subjects. For example, dogs are randomly assigned to three surgical groups for repair of rupture of the cranial cruciate ligament, and the outcome measure is peak vertical force (PVF; the maximum force applied to the ground during stance phase on the lame leg) at 6 months after surgery. ANOVA would be used to compare the group means. If the associated P value is small, at least one group mean is statistically different from the others. A limitation of ANOVA is that it does not tell you which means are different from the others. Therefore, ANOVA is usually followed by post hoc tests, a series of pairwise t tests that describe exactly which groups are different from the others. There is danger of type I error inflation in doing pairwise tests, which is described in following sections.

6. The fallacy of normal data distributions for *t* tests and ANOVA

There are several assumptions underlying *t* tests and ANOVA. The one that most people remember is the assumption of normality; that is, the data need normal distributions within groups. Normality of data is not as much of a problem as it is often perceived to be because it is the test statistic that must have the correct distribution (eg, Student's *t* distribution). If the sample size is large, statistical theories of large numbers "take over" and normality of data is not much of a problem. When the data are clearly not normally distributed, other statistical methods are available. Examples include Wilcoxon tests and nonparametric ANOVA.

Note that there are other assumptions underlying *t* tests and ANOVA that are more important than normality, for example, independence of observations and equal variances across groups.

7. What is type I error?

There is a formal statistical definition, but it is essentially concluding that a result is statistically significant when the truth is otherwise. This error is considered serious because it is anticonservative; the researcher states that the results are statistically significant (ie, "real") when they are not. Type I error may occur from an artifact with the data; however, it occurs more often when several independent groups are analyzed in pairwise fashion, each at a .05 significance, without using a type I error correction method, such as the Bonferroni correction.

There are two classic examples of "inflating the type I error rate" to greater than .05. First, a researcher has several independent groups of subjects and analyzes each pair of groups separately using the .05 cutoff, concluding that a pair of groups is statistically different if their associated *P* value is less than .05. The second example is comparing repeated measures at each time point; that is, two groups (or more) of subjects are followed over time, and statistical tests to compare groups are performed at each time point, ignoring the other time points. This is a standard approach but generally not the best one. The problem is that the repeated *t* tests are related (over time); however, that relation is unknown, and the *P* values cannot be adjusted accurately. It is also often awkward to have *P* values that are intermittently greater than and less than .05 when the data show a clear pattern that does not seem to agree with the *P* values.

A common method of avoiding the series of repeated tests is to use repeated measures ANOVA, which returns a single *P* value, and thus is not subject to type I error inflation.

8. What is the Bonferroni correction?

Researchers want the type I error (see question 5) for a study to be less than .05. This means that the chance of falsely reporting a positive result is less than 5% over the entire study. Statisticians call this the "family-wise" error rate. If more than one statistical test is performed, however, the chance of making a type I error increases over the study. For example, suppose that a study has four groups, and they are analyzed in a series of six pairwise *t* tests. The chance of making a type I error is then inflated to 26%.

The Bonferroni correction is a method of selecting a new cutoff, instead of .05, that reduces the study-wise type I error rate. It is defined as the old *P* value cutoff (usually .05) divided by the number of statistical tests. For four groups, the number of statistical tests would be six; thus, the new cutoff for statistical significance is $.05/6 = .0083$; that is, the pairs of group means are not statistically different unless the *P* values are less than .0083 rather than less than .05. The overall error rate is then controlled at .05.

9. What is type II error?

Type II error is concluding that a result is not statistically significant when the truth is otherwise. The result usually works against the researcher and is relatively common in veterinary research. The reason why is that type II error is intimately related to statistical power, which, in turn, is related to sample size. Veterinary research is often hindered (relative to human medical research) by lack of funding. This often limits the number of subjects in the study. The authors tell researchers, "If you have to ask about the number of subjects required for analysis, you can't afford enough of them."

10. What is power?

The power of a study is the probability of making the correct statistical inference, that is, the probability of correctly concluding that group means are different when they are different. Power is linked to sample size, because, intuitively, the probability of making a correct inference is much better with an extremely large sample size than with an extremely small sample size. Large power is good, and studies are often designed to have 80% power.

11. How does the reported sample size affect the study?

Sample size is a far more complicated feature of a study than most realize. It affects the power of a study; in the context of differentiating group means (eg, a *t* test, see question 4), you can always get statistical significance if the sample size is large enough and the population means are not identical. It also affects the generalizability of the study: are the study results generalizable to a larger population? Small sample sizes probably miss some of the variability present in a population, making it harder to generalize the results.

The problems with simply using a large sample size are that subjects are often expensive and hard to obtain and the resulting clinical significance may be small. The intuition behind the effect of sample size is as follows. Imagine you measure an outcome with large variability; that is, the values are widespread in the sample. It would take a large sample size to "pin down" the sample average to one that you are comfortable believing. Conversely, the average of a sample of tightly clustered values would be reliable with only a small sample. For example, you measure the weights of all horses that enter the hospital horse barn for a month. The range is quite large, because foals, miniature horses, saddle horses, and adult draft horses are admitted. It would take a large sample size to pin down the average monthly weight of horses. If you restricted the sample to Quarter Horses, however, fewer horses are needed, because the range of weights is much smaller.

What sample size is too small? Not every study needs to be inferential, that is, needs a P value. Descriptive studies provide information for future studies and can provide some insight for therapy. When P values are greater than .05, it has become fashionable to use the data collected to calculate post hoc power and then interpret the data in the context of low power. Hoenig and Heisey [3,4] discuss some problems with interpreting post hoc power. Also, distributional assumptions required by statistical tests cannot be verified with small sample sizes, and using statistical methods that are robust to departures from assumptions should be considered.

Researchers may report a prestudy sample size calculation. Be aware that sample size calculations require assumptions about the expected differences and variability of data that the researchers have not yet collected. This is often provides a "catch-22" [5] problem for researchers; if they knew that kind of information, they would not need do the study. So, sample size calculation can be influenced by researcher bias.

In production animal studies, data are often collapsed over clusters (eg, farms); in experiments, data are combined over replications that increase the sample size. It is desirable for the researcher to comment on the influence of the clusters or repetitions on the inferences. Litters, pens, and farms are all ways in which animals are naturally grouped and are examples of cluster effects. Those effects induce a correlation structure on the data that must be accounted for in analysis, because the effective sample size induced by the correlated data is smaller than the actual sample size.

12. Why do papers report several sample sizes?

The abstract for a paper and the body of a paper may report different sample sizes. Abstracts are notoriously different from the actual body of the paper. Usually, the abstract fails to describe subjects that drop out of the study, and these constitute missing data. There are two issues with missing data: the mechanism by which they went missing and how to handle the missing data in the analysis. If the data are missing completely at random (eg, the technician in histopathology laboratory lost some slides), the missing data can be ignored in the analysis without causing bias. If the missing data are related to the outcome, however, the results of the study could be biased. For example, suppose that some dogs do not return for a final 6-month follow-up and gait assessment during an orthopedics study. It may be that these dogs are all doing so well that the owners did not feel the need to return. By omitting those subjects, the study is biased.

The analysis of missing data is rich with statistical methodology, but most of it is sophisticated. Should observers be blinded when assessing objective outcome measures?

13. What are the effects of historical controls on a study?

Using historical controls instead of concurrent controls significantly weakens the impact of a study. That is because concurrent controls are subject to the same "background" effects as the experimental subjects during a study, thereby reducing bias. Controls measured last year may not have the same technicians or equipment, for example, and the study is then "comparing apples with oranges." Sometimes, for cost or ethical reasons, historical controls are preferred. In such instances, every effort should be made to justify why they are acceptable in terms of minimizing bias; that is, why they had the same experimental conditions as subjects in the current study.

14. Did the researchers appropriately randomize subjects to groups, and why is that important?

Convenience or ad hoc group assignments are not randomization techniques and can weaken the evidentiary value of a study. For example, taking half the rats out of a box and assigning them to one group while assigning the remaining half to another group is not randomization. The problem is that easy-to-catch rats are in one group, and they may be younger and smaller than fast rats. Age is a feature that may bias the study. Randomization is a way to control bias in studies by keeping confounders balanced across groups of large sample size. For small groups, blocking on known confounders can help to reduce the change of bias.

It is not always necessary or practical to do simple randomization, and alternating treatments among livestock as they pass through a chute (sequential allocation) may be an acceptable method of assigning subjects to groups. There are many other useful and acceptable variations on simple randomization that enable researchers to control variability or ensure balance of confounders across groups.

A large enough sample size randomization should control for confounding variables among groups. In companion animal veterinary medicine, it is often the case that sample sizes are small. Randomization may not have balanced confounders across groups, and it is important to compare the distributions of variables among the groups on known confounders. Sometimes, to ensure the balance of confounding variable among groups, summary statistics of confounding variables are used to compare groups. For example, sample averages may be used to verify that groups are balanced on subject weight. Data summaries do not completely describe data distributions, however, and can miss important differences among groups.

15. What inferences can be made with an experiment that does not have a comparison group?

Some studies omit control groups for comparisons and instead use comparisons with the subjects' own baseline values. The idea is that if subjects improve from baseline, the therapy must work. It could be the case that the subjects are improving as a result of the natural course of the disease or because they are receiving adjuvant care better than they would normally have (eg, more nutritious food at the hospital) in their home setting, however. Therefore, a comparison group is almost always required to show efficacy. The control group does not necessarily have to be negative controls, however; it could be a standard-of-care therapy. For example, in an analgesia study, it may not be ethical to give subjects placebo control; instead, they would be administered the standard-protocol analgesia.

Subjects can be control and experimental subjects in crossover designs. The subjects are dividend into groups, treated for a time, and, after a washout period, switch treatment groups. This design is useful when subjects can quickly (usually within days) revert to their previous state after treatment is withdrawn. Pain studies commonly use crossover designs.

16. What is standard deviation (SD) and standard error (SE)?

Both are measures of variation. The SD is roughly interpreted as the average distance of the subjects' outcome values to the sample average. Therefore, SD is a measure of sample variation, which is an estimate of population variation. The SE is the variation of a statistic (eg, means, medians). Consider the following hypothetical experiment. You randomly sample 10 horses 50 times from a population (ie, 50 samples with a sample size of 10), measure their body weight, and calculate 50 sample averages, 1 for each sample. The averages come from different samples, so they would all be different; that is, the averages have variation. The SD of the 50 averages is called the SE. It is never feasible to sample a population 50 times; thus, there are formulae used to calculate SE. Use the SD when you want to describe the variation of a sample, and use the SE to describe the variation of a summary (eg, average) of the population. Note that for averages, the SD and SE are intimately linked: $SE = SD/sqrt(N)$, where N is the sample size and sqrt() is the square root.

17. Some papers report medians instead of averages; what is the correct associated measure of variation with these statistics?

When a sample has a symmetric distribution, the average and median are the same. As the distribution of the sample becomes skewed, the average follows the longer tail of the distribution. For example, a sample of 200 Quarter Horse weights would probably be fairly symmetric, and the average and median would be approximately the same. If the 50 largest Quarter Horse weights are replaced with draft horse weights, the average would increase to reflect the influence of the weights but the median would not, because half of the subjects are always smaller than the median and half are larger (the definition of median). If the sample is skewed, the median may be a more sensible statistic to report than the median. It is difficult to calculate the SE of a median; thus, it is usually reported with a range to indicate variation. For example, a result of horse weights may look like 1005 (900, 1200), where 1005 is the median and the numbers in parenthesis are the 5% and 95% percentiles or a similar quantity.

18. How do I interpret plots: scatter plots, box plots, and histograms?

There are three common plots: scatter plots, box plots, and histograms. Plots should not be used for inference but for data description. This is because the arrangement of the axis and the choice of scale of the plot data can affect the appearance of the plot.

Scatter plots are common to regression and correlation analysis. They are a plot of two matched outcomes and appear as a cloud of points on the graph. By "stretching" one of the axes, it is possible to correctly plot but distort the appearance of the data.

Box plots are used to compare two or more groups of data visually by plotting the median, quartiles, and ranges of the data. The important thing here is that not all statistical software plots box plots in the same way.

Histograms plot the distribution of the data by plotting a bar chart of the data. To make the bars, the data must be arbitrarily grouped into sections. The size of the grouping (large or small) can dramatically affect the interpretation of the histogram.

Sometimes, continuous data are categorized into discrete data, and tables are used instead of plots. This is acceptable, but the cut points used to discretize the data should be clearly described.

19. How do I interpret measures of agreement among observers (or diagnostic tests, for example)?

There are many ways to compare two or more measurements on the same subjects. If the data are continuous, the most common way is Pearson's correlation (r^2), which measures the strength of linear association. The drawback is that two observers can have a large correlation even though one is consistently different (by a fixed quantity). For example, comparing two ways of measuring weight, if one scale is always 10 lb more than the other, the correlation is perfect. Concordance correlation is a way of measuring correlation that directly measures agreement by accounting for additive and multiplicative effects.

For scale data, the kappa statistic (κ) is widely used to measure agreement among raters. It is calculated by adjusting the percent agreement among raters by the percent agreement that is possible by chance. The κ ranges from 0 to 1, and benchmarks can be found in several articles [6]; however, they are different than those usually considered for Pearson's correlation coefficient.

20. What is regression?

Regression is a way of understanding one variable in the presence of another. For example, the lameness in dogs can be assessed with the maximum force applied (by the lame leg) to the ground during stance phase (PVF). The velocity at which the dogs moved also affects PVF; the faster the walk, the larger is the PVF. When PVF is measured, velocity is also measured, and the two can be graphed with a scatter plot. Regression analysis fits an optimal line (but could fit curves) to the cloud of points. The line is the mean PVF for every value of velocity. The slope of the line represents the effect of velocity on PVF. A large (negative or positive) slope would suggest that PVF is strongly affected by velocity, and a slope near zero suggests that there is no relation between PVF and velocity. The *P* values associated with regression test the intercept and slope of the line against zero. Small *P* values indicate that the coefficients are not statistically different from zero.

Subtracting the line from every value of PVF provides the residuals, which are PVF adjusted for velocity.

21. What are the assumptions for a statistical test?

Every statistical test and model have underlying assumptions that are required for validity. Most basic textbooks (eg, [3]) list assumptions for statistical tests, but most statistical software does not automatically verify assumptions. These assumptions should be verified during the data analysis process, but it is not always possible to describe the verification process in a paper.

References

[1] Jacobson NS, Truax P. Clinical significance: a statistical approach to defining meaningful change in psychotherapy research. J Consult Clin Psychol 1991;59(1):12–9.

[2] Sterne JA, Smith GD. Sifting the evidence—what's wrong with significance tests? Br Med J 2001;322:226–31.

[3] Ramsey FL, Schafer DW. The statistical sleuth: a course in methods of data analysis. North Scituate (MA): Duxbury Press; 2002.

[4] Hoenig JM, Heisey DM. The abuse of power: the pervasive fallacy of power calculations for data analysis. Am Stat 2001;55:19–24.

[5] Heller J. Catch-22. New York: Simon and Schuster; 1955.

[6] Landis JR, Koch GG. The measurement of observer agreement for categorical data. Biometrics 1977;33:159–74.

Vet Clin Small Anim 37 (2007) 487–497

VETERINARY CLINICS
SMALL ANIMAL PRACTICE

SEVIER
UNDERS

Critically Appraising Studies Reporting Assessing Diagnostic Tests

Annette O'Connor, BVSc, MVSc, DVSc*,
Richard B. Evans, PhD

Veterinary Diagnostic and Production Animal Medicine,
Iowa State University College of Veterinary Medicine, Ames, IA 50011, USA

This article has two sections. The first part introduces fundamental concepts critical to the evaluation of diagnostic tests. The topics covered in this section include (1) characteristics of useful diagnostic tests, (2) types of diagnostic tests, (3) outcomes from diagnostic tests, and (4) a glossary of terms used to describe the accuracy of diagnostic tests. This section does not contain any more than the most basic methods of calculation, because numerous veterinary and medical texts and Web sites already cover this information [1–3].

The second section details how clinicians should evaluate studies and their own clinical experience about diagnostic tests. The section uses a checklist published by Whiting and colleagues [4] as a means of describing the essential features of studies reporting diagnostic test accuracy. That article was published simultaneously in various medical journals and is freely available [5]. The checklist is routinely called the quality assessment of diagnostic accuracy studies (QUADAS) statement.

Although diagnostic tests can be applied for a variety of questions other than disease occurrence, such as the likelihood of a client returning for a follow-up visit, for the remainder of this article, the authors assume that most readers are interested in tests that apply to the diagnosis of disease.

DIAGNOSTIC TESTS: BASIC CONCEPTS AND GLOSSARY OF TERMS

The characteristics of a useful diagnostic test are defined by Pepe [2] as follows:

1. The disease should be serious or potentially so.
2. The disease should be relatively present in the target population.
3. The disease should be treatable.
4. Treatment should be available to those who test positive.

*Corresponding author. *E-mail address:* oconnor@iastate.edu (A. O'Connor).

0195-5616/07/$ – see front matter
doi:10.1016/j.cvsm.2007.01.007

5. The test should not cause harm to the individual.
6. The test should accurately classify diseased and nondiseased individuals.

Types of Diagnostic Tests

Diagnostic tests are varied. Practitioners are familiar with tests associated with submission of clinical specimens, such as biochemistry profiles, function tests, antibody level tests, or necropsy samples. It is less common to consider that most aspects of the clinical examination are diagnostic tests. For example, in the attempt to diagnose a condition, a practitioner may perform palpation of the abdomen and ask questions about dietary habits. All these tests have a sensitivity and specificity; however, they are rarely considered or reported.

Screening Versus Diagnostic Tests

Diagnostic tests can also be divided into screening and diagnostic tests. Screening tests are used in healthy animals and tend to be inexpensive and noninvasive. It is common for positive outcomes from screening tests to be followed up with a more accurate, expensive, or invasive test. In the context of food animals, screening tests are associated with infectious disease control and eradication programs. In the small animal setting, many aspects of a thorough clinical examination are screening tests; for example, palpation of the abdomen of enlarged kidneys in cats during a physical examination is an example of a inexpensive, imperfect, and noninvasive screening test for renal disease, and a positive finding, such as an enlarged or irregular kidney, may lead to a more expensive and invasive test. Diagnostic tests are thought of as being used in the setting of an unhealthy animal to confirm a diagnosis. Statistical issues of validation apply equally to screening and diagnostic tests.

Types of Test Results

The results from diagnostic tests can be described as categoric or continuous. Categoric test results place patients into mutually exclusive groups. Test results that include only two mutually exclusive groups are referred to as binary or dichotomous results (eg, positive or negative, present or absent, male or female animal). Multicategoric test results mean that patients fall into one (and only one) of several categories. For diagnostic tests associated with disease outcomes, multicategoric test results often have an implied order that conveys the increasing severity of disease (eg, scales or grades for hip dysplasia in dogs, body condition scores for dogs) [6]. Test results with an implied order are referred to as ordinal test results.

Diagnostic tests can also return a continuous number as the result, for example, of a red blood cell count or glucose level. These tests are invariably subject to a threshold that practitioners use as a cutoff level for decision making, with patients above a threshold level being considered disease-positive and patients below a certain cutoff level being considered disease-negative. A continuous outcome may also be converted to a multicategoric outcome. Patients with test results above a threshold cutoff level are declared positive, patients with results below a different cutoff level are declared negative, and patients with a result between the positive and negative cutoffs are suspect. The Kirby-Bauer method of describing antimicrobial resistance is an example of this approach, in which the size of the zone of inhibition is used to categorize the bacteria as susceptible, moderately susceptible, or resistant [7].

Glossary of Terms

Gold standard: a reference standard or diagnostic test for a particular illness that can perfectly discriminate positive and negative animals

Sensitivity: the probability of the test finding disease among those who have the disease or the proportion of patients with disease who have a positive test result: Sensitivity = True Positives/(True Positives + False Negatives)

Specificity: the probability of the test finding no disease among those who do not have the disease or the proportion of patients free of a disease who have a negative test result: Specificity = True Negatives/(True Negatives + False Positives)

Positive predictive value (PPV): the proportion of patients with a positive test result who actually have the disease: PPV = True Positives/(True Positives + False Positives)

Negative predictive value (NPV): the proportion of patients with a negative test result who do not have the disease: NPV = True Negatives/(True Negatives + False Negatives)

Likelihood ratio: the likelihood that a given test result would be expected in a patient with a disease compared with the likelihood that the same result would be expected in a patient without that disease

Likelihood ratio positive (LR+): the odds that a positive test result would be found in a patient with versus without a disease (Table 1): LR+ = Sensitivity/(1 − Specificity)

The probability of a test result being positive in a person with the disease divided by the probability of a test result being positive in a person without the disease: LR(+) = [TP/(TP + FN)]/[FP/(FP + TN)], where TP is true positive, FN is false negative, FP is false positive, and TN is true negative.

Likelihood ratio negative (LR−): the odds that a negative test result would be found in a patient without versus with a disease: LR− = (1 − Sensitivity)/ Specificity

The probability of a test result being negative in a person who has the disease divided by the probability of a negative test result in a person who does not have the disease: LR(−) = [FN/(TP + FN)]/[TN/(FP + TN)]

CRITICALLY APPRAISING STUDIES REPORTING DIAGNOSTIC TEST ACCURACY

Practitioners use diagnostic tests routinely, and just as therapeutic choices can be based on the best available evidence, the choices and the interpretation of diagnostic tests can be evidence based. Numerous articles report the test characteristics of diagnostic tests, but many of these studies are poorly executed and provide biased estimates of the test characteristics. Just as well-executed randomized clinical trials provide valuable evidence to support therapeutic decisions in practice, research results from well-executed comparisons of

Table 1
Determination of Sensitivity and Specificity

		Disease		
		Positive	Negative	
Test	Positive	True positive (TP)	False positive (FP)	TP + FP
	Negative	False negative (FN)	True negative (TN)	FN + TN
		TP + FN	FP + TN	

Sensitivity = TP/(TP + FN).
Specificity = TN/(FP + TN).
PPV = TP/(TP + FP).
NPV = TN/(FN + TN).

diagnostic tests can provide valuable information to the clinician about the application and interpretation of diagnostic tests.

For randomized clinical trials, guidelines, such as the Consolidated Standards of Reporting Trials (CONSORT) statement, are available to provide clinicians and researchers with minimum standards for conducting, reporting, and appraising the evidentiary value or methodologic quality of randomized trials, and similar statements are available for studies of diagnostic accuracy. The CONSORT statement was initially published in 1996 and is available [8]. The CONSORT statement is described as follows [8]:

> . . .an important research tool that takes an evidence-based approach to improve the quality of reports of randomized trials. The statement is available in several languages and has been endorsed by prominent medical journals such as *The Lancet, Annals of Internal Medicine,* and the *Journal of the American Medical Association.* Its critical value to researchers, health care providers, peer reviewers and journal editors, and health policy makers is the guarantee of integrity in the reported results of research.
>
> CONSORT comprises a checklist and flow diagram to help improve the quality of reports of randomized controlled trials. It offers a standard way for researchers to report trials. The checklist includes items, based on evidence, that need to be addressed in the report; the flow diagram provides readers with a clear picture of the progress of all participants in the trial, from the time they are randomized until the end of their involvement. The intent is to make the experimental process more clear, flawed or not, so that users of the data can more appropriately evaluate its validity for their purposes.

Similar guidelines, checklists, and flow charts are available for reporting and evaluating diagnostic tests [4,9].

For researchers, these guides provide a means of reducing the introduction of bias in the study results. For reviewers of studies, the guide specifically designed for diagnostic test evaluation should enable identification of comparisons of diagnostic tests that are susceptible to bias [10]. The introduction of bias results in the overestimation or underestimation of the sensitivity or specificity of the test (ie, the study incorrectly describes the accuracy of the test). More than 33 guidelines/checklists are available for evaluating diagnostic tests, and the 2 common guidelines/checklists are the standards for reporting diagnostic accuracy (STARD) [9] and the QUADAS [4]. The authors next discuss questions asked by the QUADAS statement, explain how they attempt to identify potential areas of bias in studies, and provide small animal–associated veterinary examples when possible. Throughout this section, the reference standard refers to the baseline or standard test, which is usually a "gold standard" or commonly used test. The index test refers to the "new" method being evaluated.

The QUADAS is a 14-question instrument tool. The questions are presented exactly as presented in the article.

1. Was the spectrum of patients representative of the patients who will receive the test?

    Do the demographics of your clients differ greatly from the patients for which you plan to use the test? For example, if the study population is dogs and you intend to use the test in cats, the results of the tests, sensitivity, and specificity may differ. For instance, antigen tests for heartworms are the gold standard antemortem test for diagnosing heartworms in dogs. Because unisex infections consisting of only male heartworms or symptomatic immature infections are more common in cats, however, antigen tests have a lower sensitivity to detect heartworm disease in cats [11,12].

    To assess the question correctly, it is important to consider demographic information, such as region, local diseases, age, breed, gender, severity of disease, and opportunity for concurrent disease. To answer this question, consider whether your patients would have been eligible for inclusion in the study. If your answer is "yes" and further evaluation of the data reveals no major biases, this implies that the test characteristics, such as sensitivity and specificity, reported in the study should be similar in your patients. If it seems unlikely that your clients could have been included in the study, the results are likely not relevant and a busy clinician may need to read no more of the study.

    Because this question does not address issues associated with internal validity (ie, study design execution), this does not mean that the study is not ultimately going to be found to provide high-quality diagnostic test evaluation.

2. Were selection criteria clearly described?

    Selection criteria refer to who was included and excluded deliberately from the study population. The study should fully disclose who was able to enter the study. This is closely related to the previous question, because the selection criteria need to be described for a practitioner to determine if the population is relevant. The selection criteria matter, because the sensitivity and specificity of diagnostic tests change for subpopulations. For example, a study reporting a new radiographic pose may have been limited to small dogs, because the pose may be difficult to achieve for large dogs. Consequently, the test characteristics, such as sensitivity and specificity, relate to small dogs, and practitioners may expect different results in large dogs. Other information that should be reported includes the start and end dates of the study, the setting (eg, private clinic, university setting), and the location.

DeFrancesco and colleagues [13] describe a group of cats with heartworm disease that variously received echocardiography, antigen or microfilaria testing, or postmortem evaluation to confirm disease status. Sixty animals defined by the reference standard had heartworm disease; however, only 43 received echocardiography. Therefore, it is not clear if the results of the echocardiography influenced the reference testing received and why this population was chosen to receive the echocardiography. It is possible that the 43 cats that received echocardiography differed in a meaningful way from the 17 cats that did not receive echocardiography; therefore, selection bias may have occurred. Factors that should be included in the description of selection criteria include the following:

- Patient recruitment procedures
- Patient demographics
- Patient and specimen inclusion/exclusion criteria
- Specimen collection procedures
- Time of specimen collection and testing
- Types of specimens collected
- Number of specimens collected and tested and number discarded
- Number of specimens included in final data analysis
- Specimen collection devices (if applicable)
- Specimen storage and handling procedures

It is also critical in this section to ensure that the populations for determining sensitivity and specificity are appropriate. The inclusion criteria for diseased and nondiseased animals should be the same. It would be inadequate, for example, to use hospital dogs for the disease-positive population and shelter dogs for the disease-negative population for determining the sensitivity and specificity of heartworm diagnostics.

3. Is the reference standard likely to correctly classify the target condition?

The reference standard refers to the test used to determine the presence or absence of the outcome of interest, and the index test is the new method of diagnosing being investigated. The reference test refers to the current gold standard, which is a test considered to the 100% sensitive and 100% specific. The sensitivity and specificity of the index test are then compared with that reference standard. Necropsy-based confirmation of the presence of heartworm disease is an example of a true gold standard test. Often, the reference standard may be known to have less than perfect sensitivity and specificity, and in this case, it is only possible to calculate the relative sensitivity and specificity. It is important to realize that a comparison of two tests in which neither is a gold standard is a measurement of agreement. Both tests could agree about a patient's status; however, compared with a gold standard, both may be wrong. There are statistical methods for estimating sensitivity and specificity when no gold standard exists, and these should be preferred over "relative" sensitivity and specificity [14–16]. Authors should acknowledge the limitations of estimates of relative sensitivity and specificity. For the diagnosis of heartworm infection in dogs, tests for antigens to *Dirofilaria immitis* are referred to as the antemortem gold standard [11,12]; however, studies using this reference standard are truly reporting relative sensitivity and specificity. For dogs, this may represent a minor difference, because less than 1% of infections are apparently patent and not antigenemic. In cats, however, the difference between antigenic test results and necropsy findings is likely larger [12].

4. Is the time period between the reference standard and the index text short enough to be reasonably sure that the target condition did not change between the two tests?

The reference test and the index test should be run on the same patients at the same time; however, there is often a delay in testing. This question requires the reader to assess whether the disease status, including severity, is the same at both time points of observation. For chronic diseases, such as cancer, a difference of days is unlikely to be significant, although weeks and months may be important. For infectious diseases, days may make significant changes in the presence of antigens and antibodies; therefore, a time delay of days between tests may introduce a significant bias in the estimate of the sensitivity and specificity of the index test. Delays longer than a few days would be inappropriate for a comparison between reference and index tests for *D immitis*, because infections may be more detectable as the worms mature.

5. Did the whole sample or a random sample of the sample receive verification using the reference standard?

If only a select subgroup received the reference test, this may lead to partial verification bias. If only a subset is chosen, it is essential that the authors mention that the sample was randomly chosen and preferable if they describe the methods of randomization. Partial subset testing occurs commonly in retrospective studies. For example, the researchers may examine hospital records and include all cases using the index test; however, only inconclusive index test cases received the reference test. In this situation, the sensitivity and specificity do not apply to all animals tested with the index test, likely a broad spectrum of the disease, but only the select subset that receives the test. Another example of partial verification bias occurs when only extreme cases are subject to the reference test (ie, clearly positive cases, clearly negative cases); again, the sensitivity and specificity reported likely are not applicable to the full spectrum of disease. If an index test for heartworm infection is only compared with the reference test when the animals have a heavy burden of microfilaria, the results may not reflect the sensitivity and specificity for prepatent infections.

It is important that the index test does not influence the decision to perform the reference test, because this leads to selection bias. This question applies only to studies that use the index text before the reference standard. Begg [10] discusses verification bias as one of the most common biases seen in diagnostic test evaluation in human literature.

6. Did the patients receive the same standard reference regardless of the index test used?

There are many circumstances in which, for a variety of reasons, the standard reference is not exactly the same for all animals in the study. The differences in the reference standard used for positive and negative animals is referred to as differential verification bias [4]. This situation occurs when reference tests are applied after the index test. The result of index testing results in the application of a more expensive, perhaps more sensitive test, whereas negative index test results are followed up with an alternative test. For example, if researchers evaluating a new antigen test for heartworm disease (the index test) used a standard antigen test as a reference standard for index test–negative animals but index test–positive animals received echocardiography and the standard antigen test as the reference, test differential verification bias might occur. A bias occurs because more "effort" is placed on verifying the animal's positive disease status than on the negative disease status (or the reverse).

A different reference standard may also be applied to all positive or negative animals if the reference standard requires training; therefore, if the sensitivity and specificity of the reference standard improve with training, this results in verification bias. A common situation in which this may occur is the use echocardiography for diagnosis of heartworm infection. In this situation, the sensitivity and specificity are likely to be lower at the start of the study and higher at the end, and the average results are reported. A clinician should be aware that the test may be less accurate initially than reported in the study. Another setting in which the reference standards may differ is studies using several clinicians or technicians to perform the reference test. Each clinician or technician may have different skills, and thus different sensitivities and specificities; again, the average is reported. It is possible to conceive of a situation occurring in which several clinicians starting with different sensitivities and specificities complete the study with different sensitivities, such that a different reference standard was used at each time by each clinician.

7. Was the reference standard independent of the index test (ie, the index test did not form part of the reference standard)?

When the result of the outcome of the index test is included in establishing the final diagnosis, this represents incorporation bias and results in bias attributable to correlation of the index test with the reference standard. An example of incorporation bias might be a study investigating force plate compression forces for the diagnostic test for soundness in dogs and using radiographic results, force plate compression forces, and the results of a physical examination to define soundness (ie, the reference). This is incorporation bias, because the index test (compression forces) is included in the reference test. If the compression force information was omitted from the reference test, this would not represent a source of bias. This form of bias can only occur when multiple tests are combined to verify the disease status and the reference standard is included in this combination of tests. In a study on evaluation of the use of echocardiography for the diagnosis of heartworm disease in cats, DeFrancesco and colleagues [13] report that the "diagnosis was confirmed in 60 of 69 cats on the basis of positive antigen or microfilaria test results, detection of heartworms on post-mortem or echocardiographic examination," suggesting incorporation bias.

8. Was the execution of the index test described in sufficient detail to permit replication of the test?

9. Was the execution of the reference standard described in sufficient detail to permit replication of the test?

It is critical that the authors present enough detail to allow the test to be applied in other settings. Just as there are minimum standards for reporting treatment protocols in randomized clinical trials, minimum standards for reporting diagnostic tests should be included. The clinician should use the detailed information to determine if he or she can reproduce the test as described in the study. For example, the sensitivity of echocardiography for heart-worm disease is likely influenced by the quality of the equipment used, and the clinician should make an adjustment for this when applying the results of the study to his or her patients.

Because of the vast array of diagnostic tests, it is not possible to list all minimum standards, but the authors provide a list of some recommended minimum requirements for reporting common types of assays. For any purchased products, the manufacturer details, including a catalog number, should be included. For in-house developed tests, all information necessary to repeat the test should be included.

I. For serology assays or biochemical tests
    A. All antigens/antibodies used in the assay, including manufacturer information.
    B. Incubation protocols
    C. Temperature changes at critical steps
    D. Wash procedures and reagents used
    E. Number, training, and expertise of the person executing and reading the index and reference standard [9]

For tests that provide a continuous outcome, the cutoff for disease levels should be defined (eg, s/p ratios for positive test results, upper and lower limits of normal ranges for biochemistry profiles). The source of the cutoff for the upper and lower limits should also be described (eg, manufacturer-recommended cutoff, normal values derived from 30 normal dogs collected 30 years ago). The report should also describe the units of the original data and any subsequent transformation.

II. For microbiology specimens
    A. Growth conditions, including broth or media
    B. Enrichment steps
    C. Incubation times and temperatures
    D. Biochemistry test used for colony identification
    E. Methods for colony picking should be described
    F. Number, training, and expertise of the person executing and reading the index and reference standard [9]

If commercial kits or media are used, the manufacturer's information and catalog numbers should be provided. For tests that provide a continuous outcome, the cutoff for disease levels should be defined (eg, zone diameters, bacterial counts). The source of the cutoff level should also be described. If there are no published guidelines and the cutoff is based on author's determination, this should be disclosed. The report should also describe the units of the original data and any subsequent transformation.

III. Questionnaires

All the questions asked should be reported, even those not associated with the outcome. Include the scales for answers (eg, yes/no, 1–5, open ended) and any system for combining the answers to create a score. The description should include the methods of application of the questionnaire (eg, interview, client left alone with the questionnaire, telephone call) and setting for the questionnaire.

10. Were the index text results interpreted without knowledge of the results of the reference standard?

11. Were the reference standard results interpreted without knowledge of the results of the index test?

This refers to blinding of the test results. This type of bias is referred to as review bias. Obviously, if the results of one test are known before determination of the results of another test, this may lead to correlation between the outcomes, and therefore improved agreement. The more subjective the test, the more susceptible test results are to this form of bias. An echocardiogram result may be influenced by knowledge that the animal has tested positive for microfilaria, resulting in an overestimation of sensitivity. If a study does not report blinding, it is most unlikely that it occurred but was not reported.

12. Were the same clinical data available when test results were interpreted as would be available when the test is used in practice?

This question is asked to ensure that interpretation of the test results in the study is the same as in the practice. For example, additional clinical information, such as age, gender, and symptoms, may affect the interpretation of a subjective test; therefore, if those data would not be routinely available in the field, the test is unlikely to work similarly in a field setting.

13. Were uninterpretable/intermediate results reported?

For some tests, the results of index testing are uninterpretable, and these results are simply removed from the analysis. The removal of uninformative results leads to an overestimation of the accuracy of the results. Bias occurs if there is an association between uninterpretable results and disease status. Studies should report the incidence of uninterpretable results and the results of the reference standard for these uninterpretable tests; this allows readers to determine if the results seem to be associated with a particular outcome, and are therefore a potential source of bias.

14. Were withdrawals from the study explained?

Patients that were enrolled in the study should complete the study; if not, the reasons for withdrawal should be described. The differences between the original study population and the final study population are important, because withdrawals may suggest that a particular subgroup differentially left the study, and thus changes the populations to which the results can be applied.

SUMMARY

The previous questions deliberately draw the reader's attention to quality issues for the evaluation of diagnostic tests. It might be tempting to use these questions to create a scoring system for passing or failing a test; however, this is not universally recommended, because the sensitivity and specificity of the questions to diagnosis a "high-quality paper about diagnostic test evaluation" have not been determined.

One issue that clinicians may have with the QUADAS checklist is the difference between study execution and study reporting, and it is true that these cannot be differentiated. Practitioners are likely to find that a large number of current articles about diagnostic test evaluations fail to address most questions. This is not surprising and has been found to be the case in reports of diagnostic tests in human medicine.

One of the major difficulties or misunderstandings about applying evidence-based medicine in veterinary medicine is the concept that lack of evidence is the basis for doing nothing; however, practitioners are required to treat animals and use diagnostic tests even when little evidence exist. The authors would suggest that practitioners treat and diagnose animals using the best information available, which usually represents a combination of literature and clinical experience; however, if that information is weak, practitioners should be cognizant that new and better information is likely to become available that would cause different practices to become more acceptable.

References

[1] Dohoo I, Martin W, Stryhn H. Veterinary epidemiologic research. Charlottetown (Canada): AVC Inc.; 2003.

[2] Pepe MS. The statistical evaluation of medical tests for classification and prediction. New York: Oxford University Press Inc.; 2004.

[3] Sackett DL. Evidence-based medicine. New York: Churchill Livingstone; 2004.

[4] Whiting P, Rutjes AW, Reitsma JB, et al. The development of QUADAS: a tool for the quality assessment of studies of diagnostic accuracy included in systematic reviews. BMC Med Res Methodol 2003;2:25–37.

[5] Whiting P, Rutjes AWS, Johannes BR, et al. The development of QUADAS: a tool for the quality assessment of studies of diagnostic accuracy included in systematic reviews. The Netherlands BMC Medical Research Methodology 2003;3:25. Available at: http://www.biomedcentral.com/1471-2288/3/25.

[6] Dorsten CM, Copper DM. Use of body condition scoring to manage body weight in dogs. Contemp Top Lab Anim Sci 2004;43(3):34–7.

[7] Prescott JF, Baggot JD. Antimicrobial therapy in veterinary medicine. 2nd edition. Ames (IA): Iowa State University Press; 1993.

[8] Available at: http://www.consort-statement.org.

[9] Bossuyt PMM, Reitsma JB, Bruns DE, et al. Towards complete and accurate reporting of studies of diagnostic accuracy: the STARD initiative. Ann Intern Med 2003;138: 40–4.

[10] Begg CB. Biases in the assessment of diagnostic tests. Stat Med 1987;6:411–23.

[11] Nelson CT, McCall JW, Rubin SB, et al. 2005 Guidelines for the diagnosis, prevention and management of heartworm (*Dirofilaria immitis*) infection in cats. Vet Parasitol 2005;133: 267–75.

[12] Nelson CT, McCall JW, Rubin SB, et al. 2005 Guidelines for the diagnosis, prevention and management of heartworm (*Dirofilaria immitis*) infection in dogs. Vet Parasitol 2005;133: 255–66.

[13] DeFrancesco TC, Atkins CE, Miller MW, et al. Use of echocardiography for the diagnosis of heartworm disease in cats: 43 cases (1985–1997). J Am Vet Med Assoc 2001;218(1): 66–9.

[14] Hui SL, Walter SD. Estimating the error rates of diagnostic tests. Biometrics 1980;36: 167–71.

[15] Alonzo TA, Pepe MS. Using a combination of reference tests to assess the accuracy of a new diagnostic test. Stat Med 1999;18:2987–3003.

[16] Dendukuri N, Joseph L. Bayesian approaches to modeling the conditional dependence between multiple diagnostic tests. Biometrics 2001;57:158–67.

Vet Clin Small Anim 37 (2007) 499–520

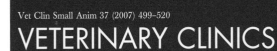

VETERINARY CLINICS
SMALL ANIMAL PRACTICE

Clinical Reasoning and Decision Analysis

Peter D. Cockcroft, MA, Msc, VetMB, DVM&S

Department of Veterinary Medicine, University of Cambridge, Madingley Road, Cambridge, CB3 OES, UK

DECISION ANALYSIS

In veterinary medicine, we often deal with greater uncertainty and weaker levels of evidence than our human medicine counterparts. We have all probably used some of the following methods when making clinical decisions:

Dogmatism: this is the best way to do it.
Policy: this is the way we do it around here.
Experience: this way worked the past few times.
Whim: this way might work.
Nihilism: it does not really matter what we do.
Rule of least worst: do what you are likely to regret the least.
Defer to experts: how would you do it?
Defer to patient: how would you like to proceed?

There are times, however, when following an explicit methodic decision-making process enables us to be more confident in the conclusion and enables us to communicate more effectively with well-informed clients and colleagues when attempting to arrive at a consensus. The application of explicit quantitative methods to analyze decisions under conditions of uncertainty is called decision analysis. When we use a methodic approach, we can also include the owner's weightings or utilities on particular outcomes. A question we should ask when making decisions is "Will the use of decision analysis identify the best course of action for the owner of my patient when two or more competing options exist?" [1].

Decision Analysis

Optimal decision making requires veterinarians to identify all possible strategies, accurately predict the probability of future events, and balance the risks and benefits of each possible action in consultation with the client. Decision analysis is a formalization of the decision-making process. The decision tree

E-mail address: expertvets@ntlworld.com

is a flow diagram outlining the outcomes that could follow each potential decision and calculates the probability and value of each event.

Situations in which decision analysis may be helpful
A condition that has multiple competing treatment options with risks and benefits may benefit from decision analysis.

- When important information may be missing (Decision analysis may identify a critical information need. This may be corrected by a literature search, or the uncertainty may still exist after a search, and this can be factored into the decision by using a wide range of reasonable subjective estimates.)
- When the owner's impact on the utilities is high
- When the risks may occur at different time points, and the impact of this needs to be explained to the owner

The method is explicit and quantitative. It forces the veterinarian to consider all the options and outcomes. The product is the best option.

Disadvantages of decision analysis
The method is time-consuming and laborious. Once a tree is made, however, it can be adapted for other patients with similar conditions. Computer programs are available to compute and draw the tree. Decision analysis cannot be performed in the absence of evidence. Going through the process can at least identify what information and level of evidence are available. This quantifies the uncertainty. Deconstructing a complex situation into component parts can help to identify the options. Owner utilities may be unrealistic, and judgment is required to guide the owner through the process.

Decision Trees
Decisions can be complex with many potential outcomes. Although human brains are good at rapidly processing many forms of complex information, we have a limited capacity to interpret competing strategies objectively with sufficient accuracy and reliability. Decision analysis provides a methodology to quantify the outcomes of decisions so that the best-informed choice, based on the best external evidence and the owner's preferred values, can be identified. An appropriate and valid decision tree is the best technique for evidence-based decision making. It recognizes the owner's value system, can be quantitatively analyzed, and makes the clinical reasoning behind a decision explicit. An audit trail of clinical reasoning is produced.

A decision tree consists of nodes that describe decisions, chances, and outcomes. The tree is used to illustrate the strategies available to the veterinarian and the likelihood of each outcome if a particular decision is made. Objective estimates of the outcomes may be derived from published research studies, records, or subjective estimates.

Decision trees are composed of the following:

• Decision nodes
Decision nodes indicate a conscious decision between two or more options. They are often depicted as squares in diagrams of decision trees.
• Chance nodes
No decisions are made at a chance node, but likelihoods are attached to each outcome derived from the chance node. The likelihoods or probabilities of the outcomes emanating from a chance node add up to 1.0 or 100%, respectively.
They are often depicted as circles in diagrams of decision trees.
• Terminal nodes
Terminal nodes are often represented as triangles or squares when no more decisions are taken. Utilities are attached to these terminal nodes to indicate the value attached to the outcome by the owner.

Utilities
Utilities use a scale from 0 to 1 that reflects how important the outcome is to the owner. They are subjective in character. The best utility is given a value of 1.0, and the worst utility is given a value of 0.0. Every other outcome receives an intermediate score reflecting its relative value to the owner when compared with the two extremes. Utility scores do not have to add up to a specific number. These values should be rational and consistent. The utility then has to be multiplied by the probability of the outcome for which it has been defined to produce the expected utility. The expected utility with the highest value is the best option. Deciding on utilities in veterinary medicine can be difficult, because the animal's welfare must be safeguarded at all costs. Nevertheless, it is important that the owner be able to express a preference. The choice of a utility is likely to be a consensus between the veterinarian and the owner.

Solving the decision tree
To identify the outcome with the highest expected utility, the probability of the terminal outcome has to be computed. This is accomplished by identifying each probability on the pathway from the terminal node to the root of the tree. These probabilities multiplied together give the probability of the outcome. If all the probabilities of the terminal nodes are added together, they should total 1.0 if likelihoods have been used or 100% if probabilities have been used. This is a useful check on mathematic accuracy. The probability of the outcome is then multiplied by the utility to compute the expected utility. In many cases, outcomes are still a matter of chance, and it is important that the owner understands that the outcome with the highest expected utility may not be achieved.

Sensitivity analysis
Sensitivity analysis is performed to establish the relative importance of particular variables. If a variable is changed, how much does it have to be changed to make a significant difference to the outcome? One-way sensitivity analysis is

when the value of one variable is changed. Two- and three-way sensitivity analyses are when two and three variable values, respectively, are changed simultaneously. When we use estimated values (eg, an estimated prevalence), sensitivity analysis is a good way of working out how accurate those estimates need to be.

Missing options
It is extremely important that options are not inadvertently omitted from the decision tree because this has an impact on the terminal outcome probabilities.

Helping owners to decide
Decision trees are effectively mathematic models that enable us to look at the final outcome arising from a particular decision (or set of decisions). The construction of a decision tree requires detailed information on the probabilities of the various outcomes and the utility of the outcome to the patient. A utility is a value that is placed on the outcome by the owner. That value may not be simply economic but may include the quality of life for the animal. The expected utility for each branch of the decision tree can be calculated from the probability of the outcome and the utility of the outcome. By examining the utilities of each terminal branch of the decision tree, the best option can be identified to optimize the patient's welfare or the owner's wishes.

The construction of a decision tree and the decision analysis proceeds according to the following steps:

1. The tree is composed of clinical decisions for which all the relevant outcomes are defined.
2. A probability is attached to each of the outcomes for the decision.
3. The probability of the terminal outcome is the product of the probabilities of the preceding outcomes.
4. A utility is attached to the terminal outcome.
5. The option with the highest expected utility is selected.
6. The effect of changing any estimated probabilities and utilities can be assessed by changing their values and observing the effect on outcome values (sensitivity analysis).

Once the tree has been constructed check that:

- All the important treatment options and outcomes of these options (good and bad) are included in the construction of the tree.
- The probabilities attached to the outcomes are based on the best evidence, and they are credible.
- The utilities are credible.
- If estimates were used, were outcome utilities generated for a credible range of values?

The quality of the decision is only as good as the estimates of the outcome probabilities and the outcome utilities. It provides patients with options that have been quantified. It also makes explicit the possible unfavorable outcomes.

Traditionally, much clinical decision making unconsciously follows the form of a decision tree but is not made explicit. By producing a decision tree, it is possible to identify the following:

- All the potential outcomes of decisions
- The patient utilities or priorities of the animal and owner
- The gaps in the data required to complete the tree

Obtaining utility values from clients and owners
Utilities represent an owner's quantitative measure for a particular outcome. The utilities that are assigned to each of the outcomes are subjective. They are not entities that we think of in numeric terms; thus, various techniques have been developed to aid their generation.

Visual analog scales. Visual analog scales have been used to assist the owner. It has been found that human beings tend to avoid placing a mark at the extremes of the scales and thereby introduce a bias.

Time trade off. The owner is presented with a trade off between the quality of life of the patient and the length of life left in time of the patient.
Consider the two health states of perfectly healthy and an impaired health status.
Assume:

$$\text{Time } (\textit{healthy}) \times \text{Utility } (\textit{healthy}) = \text{Time } (\textit{impaired}) \times \text{Utility } (\textit{impaired})$$

Time trade establishes that 4 years lived with a utility of 0.5 is equivalent to 2 years with a perfect utility of 1.0. By getting the owner to choose relative time equivalences, we are able to obtain the utility value. If the patient was faced with a potential lifetime of 4 years with a severe limp, what reduction of lifetime would you be willing to accept for the dog to have perfect health?
Assume that the owner says a reduction of 1 year (ie, 3 years without a limp is equivalent to 4 years with a limp):

$$4 - 1 \, (\textit{healthy time}) \times 1 \, (\textit{healthy utility}) = 4 \, (\textit{impaired time}) \times (\textit{impaired utility})$$

$$(\textit{impaired utility}) = \frac{(4-1)}{4} = \frac{3}{4} = 0.75$$

The utility value calculated from the owner's views on the severe limp is 0.75.

Standard gamble. In this scenario, the owner is forced to choose between accepting a certain health state for the animal or taking a gamble on a better outcome while risking the worst outcome. The owner is presented with two doors. Behind door 1 is the certain outcome for an intermediate health state for which the utility is required from the patient. Behind door 2 are two hypothetical outcomes: the best possible outcome (complete recovery) or the worst possible outcome (death). The owner has to select which door to choose. By changing the probabilities of the two outcomes behind door 2, it is possible to reach a point at which the owner finds it difficult to make a choice between door 1 and door 2. At this point, the utility is equal to the probability of the best outcome behind door 2. For example, most of us would open the second door if the likelihood of complete cure was 99.9%, and most of us would not open the second door if there were a 90% chance of death.

Decision analysis tree for therapeutic decisions
Fig. 1 illustrates a decision tree for a condition that has a surgical option and a medical option. In this example, successful surgery with no pain or deformity

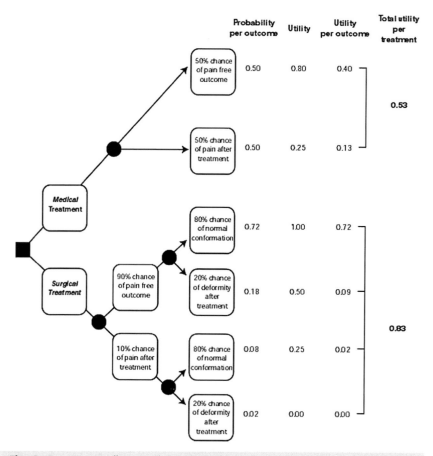

Fig. 1. Decision tree illustrates the analysis of a hypothetical decision to choose between a medical and a surgical treatment.

is the best utility (1.0), and an outcome with pain and deformity is the worst utility (0.0). Multiplying the probability of each outcome with the utility of each outcome produces the expected utility for each outcome. Adding all the medical outcomes' expected utilities together gives the expected utility of the medical option, which is 0.525 in this instance. Adding all the surgical outcomes' expected utilities together gives the expected utility of the surgical option, which is 0.830 in this instance. The conclusion is that the outcome of the surgical option is likely to be better [2].

Fig. 2 is a decision tree that was constructed to estimate the life span that might be expected for a dog presented with cryptorchidism at 1 year of age if it underwent a preventive orchidectomy or if it did not [3]. The expected utility value was expressed in terms of expected survival time in years. The decision tree indicated that there was no significant difference in the expected life

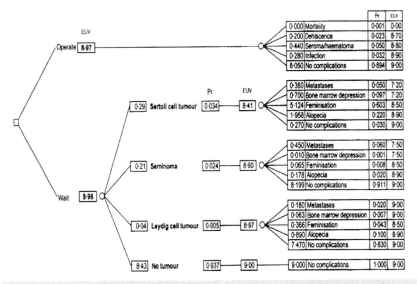

Fig 2. Decision tree for preventive orchidectomy in a cryptorchid dog. The tree has two branches: "operate" and "wait." The branch "wait" has four possibilities: "Sertoli cell tumor", "seminoma," "Leydig cell tumor," and "no tumor." The calculation of the expected utility value (EUV; expected survival time in years when the decision is made) of each branch starts on the right and proceeds to the left. The EUV of the possibilities "operate," "Sertoli cell tumor," "seminoma," and "Leydig cell tumor" are calculated by summing the products of the EUV and the probability of each possible outcome. For the branch "operate," this yields the EUV of this branch. The EUV of the branch "wait" is calculated by summing the products of the EUV and the probability of each possibility. The probabilities of "Sertoli cell tumor," "seminoma," and "Leydig cell tumor" are derived from the literature. The probability of the remaining possibility, "no tumor," is 1 minus the sum of the other probabilities in the same branch. Pr, probability, □, decision, ○, chance. (*From* Peters MAJ, van Sluis FJ. Decision analysis tree for deciding whether to remove an undescended testis from a young dog. Vet Rec 2002;150(13):409; with permission.)

span. The risk of anesthetic or surgical complications was similar to the risk of morbidity and mortality attributable to a testicular tumor. A decision tree is only a tool to help the clinician estimate the risks of treatment, and other important factors to consider before making a decision would be the behavioral changes induced by castration and the increased risk of obesity. Dog owners should be informed about these side effects. Another consideration is that cryptorchidism is considered to be inherited; thus, castration may be advisable to prevent breeding from affected animals. Because the decision tree indicated that orchidectomy would not make a significant difference to the life expectancy of the dog, it would seem advisable to monitor a cryptorchid dog frequently for the development of a testicular tumor and operate only when one is suspected.

Decision analysis tree for economic decisions
Canine gastric dilatation (gastric dilatation-volvulus [GDV]) is an acute condition affecting primarily large and giant breeds of dog. It is characterized by accumulations of gas in the stomach and varying degrees of gastric malposition leading to increased intragastric pressure, cardiogenic shock, and (often) death. Ward and colleagues [4] used a decision tree to determine the cost benefit of performing prophylactic gastropexy in the Irish Setter to avoid the condition. This is shown in Fig. 3. The expected excess expense associated with prophylactic gastropexy was US $-113.08, suggesting that the best course of action using cost alone as the outcome measure was not to perform a prophylactic gastropexy, given the current cost of the procedure. In addition to the cost outcome decision tree, a decision tree indicating the impact of gastropexy on the reduction in the lifetime probability of death from GDV (6.3% to 0.3%, a 20-fold reduction in the Red Setter) allows veterinarians and owners to make informed choices. Additional ethical issues in show animals may be other factors to consider.

Users' checklist for a decision tree analysis
    Are the results valid?
        Were all the important strategies and outcomes included?
        Was an explicit and sensible process used to identify, select, and combine the evidence into probabilities?
        Were the utilities obtained in an explicit and sensible way from credible sources?
        Was the potential impact of any uncertainty in the evidence determined?
    What are the results?
        Does one strategy result in a clinically or economically important gain?
        How strong is the evidence used in the analysis?
        Could the uncertainty in the evidence change the result?
    Are the results applicable to my scenario?
        Do the probability estimates apply to my patient or situation?
        Do the utilities reflect how my owner would value the outcomes of the decision?

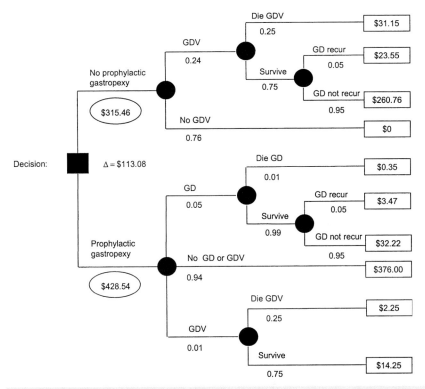

Fig. 3. Example of a decision tree for prophylactic gastropexy solved for cost for an Irish Setter (lifetime probability of GDV = 0.249). Assumptions were the cost of prophylactic gastropexy (US $400), cost of treatment for GDV (US $1500 if a dog survived and US $500 if a dog died), and cost of treatment for gastric dilatation without volvulus (US $300). (*From* Ward MP, Patronek GJ, Glickman LT. Benefits of prophylactic gastropexy for dogs at risk of gastric dilatation-volvulus. Prev Vet Med 2003;60(4):326; with permission.)

Testing and Treating Thresholds

Decision analysis can be used to decide if a patient should undergo a diagnostic test or treatment. In this analysis, the probability of disease in a patient (the pretest probability, derived from the prevalence) is compared with the testing threshold value and the treatment threshold value. Values for the following five factors are required to compute the testing and treatment thresholds:

- Benefit of therapy
- Risk or cost of therapy
- Risk of the test
- Sensitivity of the test
- Specificity of the test

The values of the benefit, risk of therapy, and risk of test can be expressed in terms of cost ($) or terms of the likelihood of a favorable outcome (0–1.0):

Testing threshold

$$= \frac{((1 - \text{specificty}) \times \text{risk of therapy}) + \text{risk of test}}{((1 - \text{specificity}) \times \text{risk of therapy}) + (\text{sensitivity} \times \text{benefit of therapy})}$$

Treatment threshold

$$= \frac{(\text{specificty} \times \text{risk of therapy}) - \text{risk of test}}{(\text{specificity} \times \text{risk of therapy}) + ((1 - \text{sensitivity}) \times \text{benefit of therapy})}$$

Whether using costs or likelihoods, the values obtained are in the range of 0 to 1.0.

The values for the testing and treating thresholds are then compared with the patient pretest likelihood (range: 0–1.0). There are three possible outcomes:

1. The probability of disease in the patient is below the testing threshold. With this result, the treatment and the test should be withheld. The risk or cost of the test outweighs the benefit of the test diagnostic information.
2. The probability of disease in the patient is between the testing and treating thresholds (the testing band). The test should be performed and treatment guided by the test result.
3. The probability of disease in the patient is above the treating threshold. Treatment should be given without testing, because the diagnostic test result is not going to change the action.

These outcomes are illustrated in Fig. 4.

General properties of testing and treating thresholds
- Testing and treating thresholds decrease as the risk of therapy decreases or as the benefit of therapy increases.
- Testing and treating thresholds increase as the risk of therapy increases or as the benefit of therapy decreases.

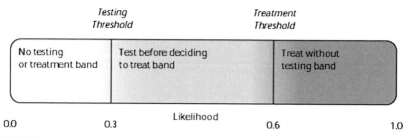

Fig. 4. Diagrammatic representation of thresholds and testing and treatment bands.

- The testing band widens as the risk of testing decreases or as the sensitivity and specificity increase.
- The testing band narrows as the risk of testing increases or as the sensitivity and specificity decrease.

Worked veterinary examples are provided by Smith [5]. Treatment and testing thresholds are covered in considerable detail by Friedland and Bent [1].

In human medicine, decision analysis has been used to provide evidence-based guidelines for patients in a defined category. These guidelines provide management strategies that deliver the highest expected utility and the lowest unfavorable outcome to patients. Although there are insufficient reliable data to enable the production of useful guidelines across a broad range of conditions, this approach could be applied to some clinical situations in veterinary medicine and, at the very least, form a basis for discussion of their potential value.

DIAGNOSTIC PROCESS

Introduction

Veterinarians make many diagnostic decisions during the course of their daily practice. The clinician should be able to explain the steps that were taken during the clinical reasoning process. Few of us are aware of the underlying mechanisms involved in making such diagnoses, however. An understanding of the diagnostic process enables information needs to be established and an audit trail of evidence-based reasoning to be realized. There are two components to the process: the identification of clinical abnormalities and disease risk factors and clinical reasoning that generates a diagnosis or differential diagnoses. They may occur, one after the other, when we arrive at a diagnosis after a complete clinical examination and taking a history, or they may be used alternately in a repeated cycle during the process of hypotheticodeductive reasoning.

Hypotheticodeductive Reasoning

Hypotheticodeductive reasoning is a highly flexible approach to problem solving. The initial hypotheses are derived from primary data acquisition. Subsequent data collection is guided by the leading hypothesis and the competing hypotheses being considered. The leading hypothesis may change depending on the new data acquired and may prompt further investigation. The competing hypotheses are compared one by one with the leading hypotheses. This process continues recursively until a critical level of confidence has been reached. The final step is usually the validation of the diagnosis. Hypothesis generation or recall is critical. A correct diagnosis cannot be made if it has not even been considered. This method produces a specific and highly efficient search for information [6]. It generates a high level of motivation in the clinician when compared with the use of a complete clinical examination as a first approach. The sign being investigated has a higher probability of being found when compared with the results of a complete clinical examination.

Diagnostic Process

Data processing is the method by which the database of information is transformed into diagnostic hypotheses or differential diagnoses. The precision of the data processing is critical. The complete or exhaustive method of data collection uses the sequence steps 1, 2, 3, and 5. The hypotheticodeductive method uses all 5 steps. The steps are as follows:

Step 1: collection of data (clinical examination, laboratory tests)
Step 2: recall of possible differential diagnoses (hypotheses)
  Hypothesis generation (recall) is an important function, because the correct diagnosis cannot be made if it is not considered. The absence of a finding common to many diseases leads to a greater reduction of the differential diagnoses than the absence of a finding specific to a single disease. Confining the search to conditions consistent with the age, gender, breed, and class of animal (signalment) also reduces the number of conditions to consider.
The recall strategies may include the recall of the following:
  • Diseases that contain all the signs observed
  • Diseases that contain only the signs you are confident about
  • Diseases for each sign
  • Diseases that contain most of the signs observed
  • Diseases that contain an important sign
  • Common diseases only
Step 3: ranking of competing differential diagnoses
  Pattern recognition is the process enabling a list of ranked differential diagnoses to be generated from the list of abnormalities. Three principle methods may be used:

  • Pattern matching
  • Probabilities
  • Pathophysiologic reasoning
Step 4: further investigations to enable differentiation of the competing hypotheses
  Go back to step 1 if there are strongly competing differential diagnoses.
  Go to step 5 if the diagnosis is confirmed as a result of evidence strongly in favor of a particular diagnosis.
Step 5: closure

These steps are illustrated in Fig. 5. Some of these steps are discussed in more detail in the following sections.

Recall and ranking

The process of recall and ranking requires a method of pattern recognition. Pattern recognition is the process leading to the generation of a list of ranked differential diagnoses from a list of abnormalities. There are three broad categories of pattern recognition: pattern matching, probabilities, and pathophysiologic reasoning.

Pattern matching. Pattern matching is a familiar cerebral process. When we notice someone, we instantly recognize a familiar face or a partially familiar face

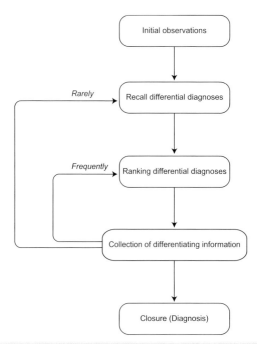

Fig. 5. Schematic representation of the diagnostic process.

or fail to recognize a stranger. The clinical signs observed are compared with profiles or descriptions of diseases we hold in our memory. The differential diagnosis list is constructed according to which of the disease profiles most closely match the clinical signs.

The pattern matching process may be restricted to common diseases in the initial hypothesis generation. If the closeness of the match deteriorates after obtaining additional data, the pattern matching may be extended to less common diseases. Pattern matching ability increases with experience, because the archive in memory is more complete and accurate.

Probabilities. A probability of a disease can be computed using the prevalence of the diseases in the population and the frequency of occurrence of the clinical signs observed within those diseases. The differential list is then constructed from the disease probabilities. The human inability to perform the mathematic computations required and the availability of data are important limiting factors.

Pathophysiologic reasoning (functional reasoning). Using the clinical signs observed, the system and the lesion within the system are identified using knowledge of disease mechanisms (pathophysiology and anatomy). A differential list is then constructed using diseases that could explain the disease processes identified. In this context, an important clinical sign is one that has an important role in the pathophysiology of the disease under consideration, which may be responsible for many of the clinical manifestations of the disease.

Which method of pattern recognition is used?
Veterinary students use pathophysiologic reasoning most often, whereas experienced veterinarians use pattern matching most often. Both groups use all three methods some of the time, and different methods may be used concurrently [7].

Clinical reasoning strategies
Sensitivity and specificity of clinical signs. Clinical signs or combinations of clinical signs all have two properties for a given disease: the specificity and the sensitivity. Sensitivity is the proportion of animals with the disease with the sign(s). Specificity is the proportion of the animals without the disease that do not have the sign(s).

The selection of a sign with a high sensitivity and specificity for a given disease can be used to confirm or rule out a diagnosis, because the sign is likely to be present if the disease is present (high sensitivity) and does not occur in other diseases (high specificity). If the sign is absent, the disease may be ruled out of further consideration. Diseases presenting clinical signs with sensitivities of 0% (common) or 100% (rare) can be eliminated from consideration if the signs are present or absent, respectively. The absence of a sign with a low sensitivity for a given disease does not rule in or rule out that disease, and therefore conveys little additional information. The presence of a sign with a low specificity does not help to differentiate the disease from other competing differential diagnoses. The presence of signs generally has a greater discriminatory power than the absence of signs. There are many more diseases with a particular sign absent than diseases with it present.

Inductive and deductive reasoning. Deductive reasoning and inductive reasoning are used alternately to investigate a hypothesis. An example of deductive reasoning is as follows: if a dog is pale, the dog may have hemolytic anemia. An example of inductive reasoning is as follows: if the dog has hemolytic anemia, the dog may have hemoglobinuria.

Abstraction and aggregation. Abstraction is a way of summarizing a group or complex of signs. Abstraction is a useful way of grouping several conditionally dependent signs together to create a finding that is more likely to be independent of other findings. In a dog, a condition comprising tachycardia (increased heart rate), tachypnea (increased breathing rate), cyanosis, and ascites could be abstracted to congestive heart failure. Similarly pale mucous membranes, tachycardia, tachypnea, low packed cell volume (PCV), and recumbency could be abstracted to anemia. By reducing the problem to a pathophysiologic description only, diseases that produce that pathophysiology need to be considered.

Prevalence. The relative prevalences of competing differential diagnoses are important information in the diagnostic process. By using broad bands of different prevalence values, it is possible to confine the initial search to diseases that are known to occur commonly.

Clinical Reasoning Checklist
To create an audit of your clinical reasoning, try to answer the following questions:

Did you follow the appropriate steps?
1. Collection of data (clinical examination and laboratory tests)
2. Recall of possible differential diagnoses (hypotheses)
3. Ranking of competing differential diagnoses
4. Further investigations to enable differentiation of the competing hypotheses
If you have evidence strongly in favor of a particular diagnosis, go to question 5.
If you are still unable to decide on a diagnosis, go to question 1.
5. Diagnosis confirmed, closure
When formulating a differential diagnosis list, did you
• Recall diseases that contain all the signs observed
• Recall diseases that contain only signs you are confident about
• Recall diseases for each sign
• Recall diseases that contain most of the signs observed
• Recall diseases that contain an important sign
• Recall only common diseases
When ranking the differential diagnosis list, which method of pattern recognition did you use?
• Pattern matching
• Probabilities
• Pathophysiologic reasoning
Which of the following strategies did you use?
• Specificities and sensitivities of clinical signs
• Logical exclusion of a disease (sign present never recorded in disease)
• Inductive and deductive reasoning
• Aggregation of clinical signs
Have you identified outstanding information needs?

CRITICAL APPRAISAL OF CLINICAL DIAGNOSTIC DECISION SUPPORT SYSTEMS
Introduction
A clinical diagnostic decision support system (CDDSS) is a system that assists a clinician with one or more component steps of the diagnostic process. Past and present CDDSSs incorporate inexact models of the incompletely understood and exceptionally complex process of clinical diagnosis. They are at

their most powerful when they provide information about one aspect of the process, allowing the clinician to form a judgment. Pattern recognition techniques are an important component in medical decision support systems and are used for the classification of a patient into a diagnostic or treatment group.

Information regarding the performance of CDDSSs is often lacking, and the output of such systems is often misunderstood. All CDDSSs should make their methodology, reasoning, and sources of information explicit. In addition, there should be a measure of their proficiency, such as accuracy or, ideally, their specificity and sensitivity. Decision support systems within veterinary science have been developed in a wide range of domains. In spite of this, their uptake and use is still low. CDDSSs for small animals have included the domains of clinical pathology, electrocardiogram (ECG) interpretation, and clinical diagnosis.

Pattern Recognition Methods

An understanding of the methodology that may be used by a CDDSS is helpful when trying to appraise the evidence being provided by a CDDSS critically. Logic, list matching, and probabilities are described with veterinary examples. Knowledge-based systems and neurologic networks that can capture relational aspects of disease are few in number and are not described; details of these can be found elsewhere [2].

Logic

Logic is an important and powerful concept in medical reasoning. For example, a disease can be excluded if a sign is observed that has never been recorded in the disease. This, of course, assumes that there is a single condition affecting the animal and that the recorded signs for a disease are accurate, complete, and absolute. In spite of these criticisms, logic still remains the most dominant pattern recognition method in a simple CDDSS. Logic forms part of list matching.

With categoric information (ie, a sign is present or not), simple algorithms consisting of a series of branching decision nodes can be devised. Example of the questions and answers encountered during the investigation of polydipsia and polyuria in a dog using the Vetstream Canis system (Vetstream Ltd, Cambridge, United Kingdom) [8] is shown in Tables 1 and 2. The system takes the user through a series of questions for which a categoric answer is required, such as absent or present and normal or abnormal. The system uses logic to retain or exclude conditions. The next question is designed to rule in or rule out diseases, producing a diminishing list of differential diagnoses.

List matching

List matching compares a patient's disease profile with stored profiles of diseases in the database. PROVIDES (canine; Impromed Computer Systems, OshKosh, Wisconsin) and Consultant (canine and feline) [9] are

Table 1

Example of the questions and answers encountered during investigation of central diabetes insipidus in a dog using Canis (Vetstream)

Question 1	Is the animal polydipsic and polyuric?	Yes
Question 2	Is there a history of recent/current medication using any of the following? Glucocorticoids Mannitol Dextrose Diuretics Phenytoin	No
Question 3	If female, is the animal 2–8 weeks postestrus and showing signs of pyometra?	No
Question 4	Have any of the following occurred? Recent exposure to high temperatures Recent extreme physical exposure Recent change in diet to dry and salty food	No
Question 5	What are the urinalysis results? Glycosuria Proteinuria Normal	Normal
Question 6	What are the findings on routine biochemistry? Decreased potassium Increased urea and creatinine Increased alkaline phosphatase Normal	Normal (potassium: 4.0–5.5 mmol/L, urea: 2.0–8.0 mmol/L, alkaline phosphatase: 10–300 IU/L)
Question 7	What are the results of the corticotropin stimulation test or low-dose dexamethasone suppression test? Both test results normal Both test results abnormal	Both test results normal
Question 8	What is the urine specific gravity? 1.001–1.006 >1.007	1.001–1.006 (normal range: 1.015–1.040)
Question 9	What is the result of the modified water deprivation test? Water deprivation test concentrating urine (specific gravity >1.025) Water deprivation test does not result in increased concentration of urine	Unable to concentrate
Question 10	How did the animal respond to antidiuretic hormone? No response to antidiuretic hormone, no increase in urine specific gravity Response to antidiuretic hormone, urine specific gravity >1.025	Concentrates urine in response to antidiuretic hormone

Table 2
Example of the differential diagnoses considered during investigation of central diabetes insipidus in a dog using Canis (Vetstream)

Differential diagnosis	Question leading to elimination
Common	
Chronic renal failure	6
Diabetes mellitus	5
Hyperadrenocorticism	7
Iatrogenic polydipsia	2
Pyometra	3
Intermediate	
Amyloidosis	5
Cystitis	5
Glomerulonephritis	5
Hepatic disease	6
Hypercalcemia	6
Hypoadrenocorticism	6
Physiologic causes of polydipsia	4
Pyelonephritis	5
Rare	
Acromegaly	5
Central diabetes insipidus	Not eliminated
Early renal failure	8
Fanconi syndrome	5
Hyperviscosity syndrome	5
Hypokalemia	6
Nephrogenic diabetes insipidus	9
Postacute renal failure	6
Primary renal failure	5
Primary renal glycosuria	5
Psychogenic polydipsia	9

two computer-based veterinary examples of list-matching diagnostic algorithms.

Consultant requires the input of a clinical sign or signs. From this, it generates the differential diagnoses, a list of diseases that produce the sign or signs. This is a simple list-matching procedure. Six signs from a case of feline hyperthyroidism were entered. The signs entered and the output from Consultant are as follows:

Species: feline
Signs entered
  Weight loss
  Tachycardia
  Polyphagia
  Polyuria
  Polydipsia
  Hyperesthesia

Possible diagnoses
  Antihistamine toxicity
  Feline infectious peritonitis
  Hyperthyroidism
  Lymphoma
  Portosystemic shunts, hepatic microvascular dysplasia

PROVIDES generates a differential diagnosis list by comparing the patient's attributes with a profile of expected findings for each disease. The system creates a list of differential diagnoses by comparing patient characteristics with patterns of discriminatory findings ("propensities") for each disease. The profile consists of findings that are strongly associated with the disease and, at the same time, tend to differentiate it from other potential causes of the patient's problems. Diseases are then ranked according to the ratio of findings exhibited by the patient to those expected for the disease. PROVIDES does not attempt to arrive at a single diagnosis but is rather intended to provide a list of reasonable possibilities for the clinician to consider. No disease is excluded just because it cannot account for all the patient's signs. An example of the output from PROVIDES for a 10-year-old dog from the southwestern United States with a chronic, intermittent, productive cough; weight loss; and lameness is shown in Table 3. Radiographs and laboratory studies have not been completed; hence, the large number of findings with no data.

Probabilities (Bayes' rule)

Canid (Animal Information Management, Victoria, Australia) is a CDDSS for dogs. It is an example of a CDDSS that uses probabilities assuming conditional independence of the clinical signs to generate a ranked list of differential diagnoses from clinical data. A probability is computed using Bayes' theorem. This theorem requires the prevalence of the diseases in the population and the frequency of occurrence of the clinical signs observed within those diseases.

Conditional independence simply means that it is assumed there is no link between the presence of an abnormality, such as a clinical sign, and other clinical signs seen in that disease. Errors occur because, pathophysiologically, signs occur together more frequently than if conditionally independent. Conditional independence of signs is assumed because the sensitivities of the sets of clinical signs within diseases are largely unknown or not reported. The frequency of occurrence of any combination of signs can be computed from the sign frequencies of the individual signs if conditional independence is assumed.

Some related systems, known as Bayesian belief networks, generate the probability of the sign(s), given that the disease is present. They do not rely on the probability of the disease being present, given the sign (s), which would need disease prevalence data. This distinction is important to understand.

Table 3
Example of the output from PROVIDES for a 10-year-old dog from the southwestern United States with a chronic, intermittent, productive cough; weight loss; and lameness

PROVIDES differential diagnosis for canine cough

Rank	Cause	Present/expected	Missing data points
1	Heartworm	3/4	5
2	Chronic bronchitis	3/4	0
3	Coccidioidomycosis	4/6	4
4	Actinomycosis	3/5	4
5	General lymphosarcoma	2/4	3
6	Pulmonary neoplasia	2/4	1
7	Laryngitis	2/4	0
8	Lymphoid granulomatosis	1/2	3
9	*Crenosoma vulpis* infection	1/2	0
10	Tuberculosis	3/7	1

Questions You Should Ask When Using a Clinical Diagnostic Decision Support System

Because the published performance indices of expert systems quoted are often difficult to interpret, or even absent, it is important that other aspects of the construction of the CDDSS are critically appraised to assess the evidence they are providing.

1. What is the source of the clinical information within the system?
   - Is it based on expert opinion?
   - Is it derived from the literature?
   - Is it derived from a database of "real" cases?
2. Is the information derived from the same population as that which I wish to use the system for?
3. If clinical sign frequencies are used, is it likely that the point of contact between the veterinarian and the sick animal is the same in my population as that used within the system? Remember, sign frequencies are different depending on the stage of disease at which the veterinarian is requested to examine the animal.
4. In addition to entering the signs I have observed, does the system enable me to enter signs I have not seen or signs I have not examined?
5. If prevalence is used, is it:
   - Expert opinion derived?
   - Obtained from cross-sectional surveys?
   - The same in my population?
   - The prevalence that is presented to the veterinarian?
   - The true prevalence of disease?
6. Do I understand how the expert system works?
7. What is the result telling me?
8. Does the expert system use a pattern recognition system based on assumptions that may make the output inaccurate? For example, if the expert system uses probabilities to generate the probability of a disease using a given set of clinical signs, is conditional independence assumed?

9. If information is provided regarding the performance of the CDDSS, do I understand what it is telling me? Accuracy is commonly used as a parameter of performance. Ideally, the specificity and the sensitivity of the system should be defined for the target population.

How has the accuracy has been assessed?
   - Using a selection of literature case reports based on availability
   - Using several cases that have subsequently been examined postmortem and a "gold standard" diagnosis obtained within a hospital environment.
   - Using several cases for which a putative diagnosis is made
   - Defined by a correct diagnosis being at the top of a list of ranked differential diagnoses and sometimes in the top five of a ranked diagnosis
   - By asking experts if the rank and probabilities produced seem to be realistic
   - By measuring the impact of patient outcomes in case-control studies
   - Using clinicians with different experience levels in different practice settings and different geographic areas to assess the impact on performance with different populations
   - By comparing the system with the performance of clinicians at different experience levels when presented with the same information

SUMMARY

Decision analysis may include the use of decision trees or audits of our decision-making process. The latter may include the use of a CDDSS. There is a time cost to perform these functions, and we have to prioritize out time budgets and select the diagnostic problem for detailed analysis with care. Nevertheless, with careful selection and appropriate critical appraisal, we can optimize the care of our patients and provide evidence-based informed choices for owners. Last but not least, we are able to justify the decisions we have made explicitly and quantify the evidence supporting them.

References

[1] Friedland DJ, Bent SW. Treatment and testing thresholds. In: Friedland DJ, editor. Evidence-based medicine: a framework for clinical practice. New York: Lange Medical Books/McGraw-Hill; 1998. p. 59–82.
[2] Cockcroft PD, Holmes MA. Decision analysis, models and economics as evidence. In: Handbook of evidence-based veterinary medicine. Oxford (UK): Blackwell Publishing; 2003. p. 154–81.
[3] Peters MAJ, van Sluis FJ. Decision analysis tree for deciding whether to remove an undescended testis from a young dog. Vet Rec 2002;. 30;150(13):408–11.
[4] Ward MP, Patronek GJ, Glickman LT. Benefits of prophylactic gastropexy for dogs at risk of gastric dilatation-volvulus. Prev Vet Med 2003;12;60(4):319–29.
[5] Smith RD. Use of diagnostic tests. In: Veterinary clinical epidemiology. London: Butterworth-Heinemann; 1991. p. 45–6.
[6] Miller RA, Geissbuhler A. Clinical diagnostic decision support systems: an overview in clinical diagnostic decision support systems. In: Berner ES, editor. Evidence-based medicine: a framework for clinical practice. New York: Springer; 1999. p. 3–34.

[7] Cockcroft PD. A survey of pattern recognition methods in veterinary diagnosis. Journal of Veterinary Education 1998;25(2):21–3.

[8] Vetstream Canis. Vetstream Ltd, Three Hills Farm, Bartlow, Cambridge, CB1 6EN, UK. Available at: www.vetstram.com. Accessed April 22, 2006.

[9] Consultant. http://www.vet.cornell.edu. Accessed April 22, 2006.

Vet Clin Small Anim 37 (2007) 521–532

VETERINARY CLINICS
SMALL ANIMAL PRACTICE

The Power of Practice: Harnessing Patient Outcomes for Clinical Decision Making

Karen Faunt, DVM, MS[a],*, Elizabeth Lund, DVM, MPH, PhD[b],
Will Novak, DVM, MBA[a]

[a]Banfield, The Pet Hospital, PO Box 13998, 8000 NE Tillamook Street,
Portland, OR 97213, USA
[b]DataSavant, 8000 NE Tillamook Street, Portland, OR 97213, USA

D ecision tree analysis, as discussed in a previous article in this issue, is a process that formalizes medical decision making so that patients benefit from veterinary care that has the highest degree of certainty of a positive outcome. Evaluation of clinical outcomes also optimizes the patient care process by transforming what is learned about a population of patients and making this information available to apply to an individual patient. As such, the practice of evidence-based medicine (EBM) relies on the ability to evaluate patient outcomes. As a result of aggregation and analysis of patient outcomes, knowledge is derived that has the potential to enhance clinical decision making and client communication. This article focuses on the processes needed to make clinical experiences in everyday practice usable and valuable to veterinary medicine as a whole.

The power of veterinary practice springs from the various encounters that occur day-in and day-out for each and every practitioner. When these encounters are examined collectively, they have the power to transform future medical decision-making practices for all veterinarians. This power is lost when records are unclear and standardized processes are not followed or when a patient's concerns are not brought to conclusion with a recorded final diagnosis and response to treatment. Establishing a diagnosis is a process of removing uncertainty until the veterinarian believes, with a high degree of confidence, that the suspected diagnosis is correct. Typically, this involves combining historical, physical, and laboratory findings. Bringing the diagnostic process to conclusion and recording it in a searchable medical record is important to the individual pet and to veterinary medicine as a whole.

*Corresponding author. E-mail address: karen.faunt@banfield.net (K. Faunt).

0195-5616/07/$ – see front matter
doi:10.1016/j.cvsm.2007.01.008

STEPS TO PRACTICE EVIDENCE-BASED MEDICINE

Becoming an evidence-based practitioner begins with awareness and understanding of the concepts and applications of EBM. How do these concepts translate into real clinical practice? The first step in the practice of EBM begins with the patient encounter and the questions and discussions about diagnosis, therapy, and prognosis. Some of these questions might include the following:

What is the best strategy to prevent obesity in dogs?
What are the risk factors for feline hyperthyroidism?
Is one treatment of flea allergy dermatitis more effective than another?
How can I communicate the certainty of this diagnosis to my client?

The second step in the EBM process is capturing the patient data acquired during the process of providing veterinary care. The recording of clinical information, ideally in a standardized fashion using common systems of nomenclature shared by other veterinarians, is essential. Becoming part of practice groups or connecting with other practices that use the same computerized practice management system can facilitate this process. Recording these data in a standardized way that is searchable is the paramount concern, however.

Efforts are underway to involve veterinarians in the third step of practicing EBM, the collection and analysis of medical outcomes for clinical research. There are many examples of successful multicenter research trials in veterinary medicine that have produced valuable information [1,2]. In Great Britain, the Cambridge Infectious Disease Consortium (CIDC) has taken this a step further by establishing an active network of motivated research-capable veterinarians working in clinical practice or practice-related roles [3]. The objective of this outreach program is to bring together veterinarians who work in practice, academia, and research and to have them work as a team. All these efforts should continue to thrive and add to the knowledge base for veterinarians.

The fourth and final step in the practice of EBM is literature review and, perhaps most importantly, the incorporation of valid clinical evidence into veterinary care. In human medicine, the Cochrane Collaboration [4] produces and disseminates systematic reviews of health care interventions and promotes the search for evidence in the form of clinical trials and other intervention studies. Also in human medicine, the organization Patient-Oriented Evidence That Matters (InfoPOEMS) generates daily electronic mail that delivers relevant and valid new clinical information from reviewed articles using specific criteria for validity and relevance to practice [5]. Similar efforts in veterinary medicine have begun. This includes the addition of veterinary references as critically appraised topics (CATs). CATs are summaries of research papers generated using strict guidelines. CATs are stored electronically in a searchable database for ease of use. By allowing all interested individuals to add to these CATs, the work of assessing outcomes is shared and could make the final step of EBM practice a reality for many veterinarians [6].

OUTCOMES

A clinical outcome is an event that follows as a result or consequence of a disease process or intervention. Outcomes are relevant observations of the disease process or clinical intervention. Clinically relevant outcomes can, for example, characterize morbidity using temperature, white blood cell count, blood urea nitrogen (BUN), and adverse reactions; record time to mortality (survival); or measure the presence or absence of disease for an individual. It is imperative that all these clinical outcomes are included in the record for further evaluation and summary if and when needed.

Once these outcomes are recorded, researchers can summarize the data for further review and analysis. Medical outcomes are used as the variables in population analyses; the type of variable determines the statistical methods that are used. For example, a white blood cell count would be a numeric variable that would be represented as a mean and compared using a t test. A proportion (percent with and without a disease) would be analyzed using a χ^2 test. Univariate analyses focus on a single variable and its relation to an outcome (eg, body condition [obesity], diabetes), whereas multivariate analyses examine the relation of many variables together to the outcome (eg, age, body condition, breed, diet, diabetes). A multivariate model allows control for confounding factors to determine the independent risk contribution for each variable. Confounding factors prevent the separate assessment of risk for each variable and occur when two variables are related to each other as well as to the outcome of interest. For example, in a study of perianesthetic morbidity and mortality in cats, duration of anesthesia was related to the preanesthetic status and to the outcome—morbidity [7]. It is not important that the individual practitioner be able to use statistical methodologies, but it is important for us all to recognize that valid research needs accurate and complete data input as well as interrogation by appropriate analytic methodologies.

With diagnostic outcomes collected from private practices, national and practice-specific disease prevalence rates can be estimated, quantifying the probability of a particular disease. Knowing the prevalence of feline leukemia virus (FeLV) infection helps to rule in or rule out the disease in a 6-year-old, male, intact Domestic Shorthair cat with decreased appetite and weight loss. Disease prevalence is the probability that an individual in a defined population is diseased before diagnostic testing. The likelihood that a result reflects a truly diseased or nondiseased condition is critical to the clinical decision-making process. In addition, the prevalence of disease in a population influences the ability of a specific test to predict whether an individual animal is truly diseased or not. If a disease is relatively common in a population, there is a higher probability that a test is able to predict a truly diseased individual (ie, there are few false-positive results). Alternatively, if a disease is relatively rare, the ability of the test to identify a truly diseased individual is diminished and more false-positive results are identified.

The knowledge gained by evaluating outcomes can help with decision making throughout the patient encounter with diagnosis, treatment, and discussing the prognosis with a client. How likely is the diagnosis of pancreatitis in a

3-year-old, spayed, female German Shepherd that has been vomiting for 24 hours and is depressed, febrile, and 5% dehydrated? If there were evidence from a population-based study that a threefold elevation in serum amylase was 11 times more likely to occur in a dog with pancreatitis than in a dog without pancreatitis, would you be more certain of the diagnosis? Alternatively, consider a 9-year-old Labrador Retriever with chronic renal failure of undetermined causes and a serum creatinine level of 3.5 mg/dL. From the results of a clinical trial [8] on the impact of dietary phosphorus restriction on survival in dogs with induced renal failure, evidence demonstrates that 8 of 12 control dogs died compared with 3 of 12 dogs in the treatment group. This information could influence your treatment plan for this pet and help to communicate the prognosis to the client. Recording these outcomes consistently for all patients and in a standardized format is critical to transforming the data from the individual into meaningful clinical information. The medical record is an essential source for the capture and ultimate retrieval of these outcomes for population analysis.

CAPTURING OUTCOMES IN PRACTICE

Communication of information is critical to the practice of veterinary EBM. Paper-based records often communicate medical information in random non-systematic ways. Computerized medical records offer veterinarians the most efficient and seamless method for capturing relevant clinical outcomes in a consistent and standardized fashion. There are many benefits to becoming a "paperless" practice. Some of these include increased organization, because data can be displayed in a variety of different ways; the ability to determine who created what information and when; improved security by limiting file access; improved legibility; and electronic transfer of digital images (eg, radiographs) and information.

In a paper-based record system, most of the information lies buried in paper files that do not lend themselves easily to aggregation and analysis. A paperless system provides faster access to needed clinical information and facilitates the ability to create portable records for patient transfers to other general and specialist practitioners as well as the maintenance of electronic records for reporting purposes to external agencies. Although there has been concern that electronic medical records have a negative impact on the patient encounter, research has not supported this concern [9]. Additionally, computerized records can be used to generate reminders that improve preventive and interventive care. Because of these and other advantages, President George Bush called for the widespread adoption of electronic health records for human patients in his 2004 State of the Union address.

One existing example is the way in which Banfield, The Pet Hospital uses its national computerized record system called PetWare (Banfield, The Pet Hospital, Portland, Oregon). This system standardizes the recording of the various components of the pet encounter, including signalment, presenting complaint by category, standardized physical examination findings (normal and abnormal; Figs. 1–3), presumptive and final diagnoses, specific diagnostics and treatments offered and provided, and searchable freehand typed additional medical notes along with financial information. Pet outcomes data recorded in PetWare are saved daily into a centralized searchable database. Outcomes data collected during pet encounters from each of the 549 Banfield hospitals are available for aggregated analysis and evaluation. As of June 2006, Banfield's database contained 34,280,033 encounter records from 6,580,149 dogs and 2,701,794 cats seen since January 1, 2001. There are other veterinary databases, but they have limitations for evaluation of outcomes for primary care practice. The Veterinary Medical Database (VMDB) contains pet records from patients seen at academic centers of veterinary medicine [10]. Because these pets are referred to teaching hospitals for care, they are likely to be atypical and not representative of patients seen in primary care settings. Another large database [11] was captured for a narrow window of time and, as such, cannot assess temporality of disease association or track changes in disease prevalence over time. Large centralized and searchable electronic medical records like this and others allow for interrogation of information that can further our knowledge base when EBM is used.

COMMUNICATION OF OUTCOMES: STANDARDIZED NOMENCLATURE

Capturing outcomes in computerized record systems is only one of the necessary components of outcomes evaluation for veterinary EBM. Communication

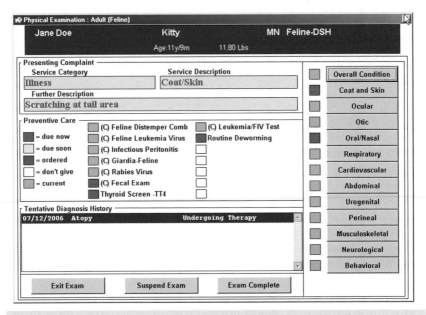

Fig. 1. Entry physical examination screen from PetWare.

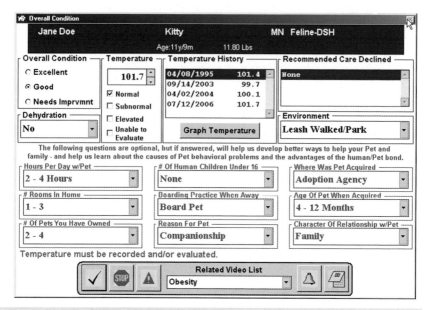

Fig. 2. Overall condition screen in PetWare.

among many record systems is essential for aggregation and analysis of medical outcomes. This communication requires the use of standardized nomenclature and a system for communication of knowledge using a controlled vocabulary of descriptive terms, with or without codes—a form of language. Written and spoken medical language, however, is not completely standardized, which is a result of nuances in semantics and the breadth of vocabulary [12]. For example, the terms *Cushing's disease* and *hyperadrenocorticism* may be used to describe the same clinical entity, and depending on an individual's medical knowledge and experience, it may not be apparent that the terms are synonymous.

The benefits of standardization of medical language include better communication and sharing of information across institutions and individuals, better recording and retrieval of information from the medical record, and increased ease of aggregation of data for an individual over time and among individuals for research and analysis [13]. In human medicine, there is a concerted effort to move to consistent nomenclature, such as systemized nomenclature of medicine (SNOMED) terms. The terms used in SNOMED have been converted to companion animal veterinary appropriate terms and are known as PetTerms [14]. These terms should be considered as a standard to adopt across companion animal practices and would improve our ability to aggregate outcomes across different practices.

It is critical that veterinarians not only be able to communicate across other veterinary practices with standardized nomenclature but across other health disciplines. The National Library of Medicine's Unified Medical Language

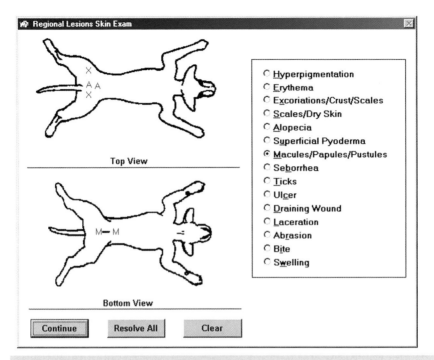

Fig. 3. Skin examination screen in PetWare; note that the doctor can place multiple notations of lesions on the ventral or dorsal body surface.

System (UMLS) has been designed to facilitate the development of computer systems that behave as if they "understand" the meaning of the language of biomedicine and health. The UMLS [15] translates disparate sources of medical data and information from many "languages," including SNOMED clinical terms (CT), medical subject heading (MeSH), and logical observation identifiers names and codes (LOINC). The outcomes data generated as a result of clinical practice, if captured, can be used to enlighten future medical decision making. To fail to capture this information from clinical encounters is to throw away clinical experience and its potential to have a positive impact on the practice of veterinary medicine.

MEDICAL QUALITY AND STANDARDIZATION OF BEST PRACTICES

Through pressures to contain costs, human medicine has been moving to standardize patient care through the application of practice guidelines and to assess outcomes of disease management. Multiple publications in human literature in the past few years document that the use of highly specific standardized treatment protocols improves outcomes for varied conditions, including treatment for postacute myocardial infarctions, care of patients undergoing detoxification therapy, and treatment for obstetric hemorrhage [16–18]. Additionally, a systematic review of evidence-based clinical guidelines in practice supports the conclusion that outcomes are improved when these types of guidelines are followed [19]. The major limitation cited by this article was a paucity of appropriate trials to review, however. Computers should play an increasing role in meeting this challenge [20]. Standardization of medical practice facilitates the measurement and comparison of outcomes that are similar, such that meaningful results are generated. If every diagnosis of Cushing's disease is based on different criteria, it can be difficult to generate meaningful estimates of disease prevalence. The same holds true for disease management. If there are not standard approaches to therapy, it can be difficult to evaluate outcomes, such as treatment efficacy or survival rates.

Protocols (best practice guidelines) are the methods by which veterinarians practice, (ie, a logical group of diagnostic tests and treatments for a specific diagnosis or presenting complaint). To measure quality, a definitive standard must be agreed on, (eg, routine or mandatory preoperative blood work). An example of how protocols can be developed and used in general companion animal practice is the use of a Medical/Surgical Protocols Standards Committee by Banfield. This committee is made up of veterinarians practicing in Banfield hospitals. Each year, they review and update all the protocols and standards of preventive, medical, and surgical procedures for the entire practice. The examination process for these protocols and standards includes a review of current literature and internal data. The standards generated are the minimum believed to be necessary to support an excellent level of general companion animal practice. These protocols and standards are operationalized through PetWare and medical practice at Banfield hospitals. Instituting a common means of practice (ie, protocols) produces outcomes data for patients that can be compared on a more universal level across an entire practice or multiple practices.

Practicing quality medicine demands that practitioners incorporate the most up-to-date and proven evidence into medical decision making. Medical knowledge is dynamic, changing as populations change and as our tools to diagnose and treat patients evolve. As new information is evaluated, it is important to remember the hierarchy of sources, wherein clinical trials and meta-analyses provide more valid evidence than case reports, editorials, or expert opinions.

As such, practicing standardized medicine does not mean that a veterinarian functions in a static way ("cookie-cutter" medicine) but quite the contrary. Practice standards and guidelines are dynamic and change as new evidence is available that supports the introduction of new diagnostic processes or therapies. These practice guidelines provide the doctor with a framework within which decisions and assessments can be made that ultimately improve patient outcomes. For example, as a result of an analysis of outcomes captured by PetWare in Banfield hospitals, a decision was made to change the disease screening protocol for FeLV and feline immunodeficiency virus (FIV). Testing for FeLV and FIV is now no longer part of the Banfield protocol for annual rechecks; FeLV and FIV testing is still performed on previously untested cats and kittens and is routine in ill cats. The decision was driven by the finding that the positivity rates of disease for screening of FeLV and FIV infection were much higher for cats that were "sick" at the time of testing versus those that were healthy. Specifically, from December 2004 to May 2005, 83,151 healthy and sick cats were tested for FeLV and FIV. Of these, 636 (0.77%) were positive for FeLV, 835 (1.0%) were positive for FIV, and 124 (0.15%) were positive for both. Additionally, 93% of the FeLV- and FIV-positive cats were considered ill at the time of testing [21]. In another analysis of the Banfield database, adverse patient outcomes within 3 days after vaccination were examined to characterize which dogs were at the highest risk for an adverse vaccine reaction based on age, breed, and gender [22]. These results can become powerful tools to communicate with clients as well as when anticipating treatment needs for dogs at risk for postvaccination reactions. Knowing the prevalence rates of disease can help to discriminate among diagnostic ruleouts on a differential list [23]. Also, from the analysis of treatment outcomes in practice, the safety and efficacy of prophylactic and therapeutic treatments can be evaluated [24]. This information is only available for evaluation through the use of a standardized electronic medical record as well as through established best practice guidelines. Although your hospital may not see the volume of cases seen at a national practice, if you set best practice guidelines and record results in a consistent searchable fashion, you can begin to develop your own information for individual use or to add to the information database of other hospitals for combined evaluation.

CRITICAL EVALUATION OF OUTCOMES

The standardized process of evaluating patient outcomes can produce a wealth of information. Within a practice, a proactive process of individual case review can be integral to outcomes assessment. This process can be as simple as establishing morbidity and mortality rounds or always recommending a full necropsy on every pet death or as complex as developing a full system to review case outcomes. Because of its unique centralized electronic medical record system, Banfield was able to establish its review process as part of its internal quality assurance program in 1987 to help ensure that only the highest standards of medicine were practiced in all Banfield hospitals. This comprehensive quality assurance program includes reviewing preventive and interventive care offered and provided to clients as well as standard review of all unexpected pet deaths through a formalized process with the doctor involved by his or her peers. As a result of these processes, Banfield captures many vital statistics about its practice, including anesthetic death rates and vaccine reaction rates for the Banfield population. Banfield is then able to share this information and is continually working to improve outcomes. Without objective consistent review of case outcomes, it is difficult or impossible to increase our knowledge base. The establishment of an internal review process can help you to direct your practices and procedures objectively.

PRACTICE-BASED RESEARCH NETWORKS

With an established network of practices in place that captures outcomes data for evaluation, the potential exists for practices to form their own research networks by region or specialty (eg, dentistry). The major advantages of practice-based research derive from the ability to study the patients to which the research results are to be applied [25–27]. A large number of pets, especially for prevalent diseases, can be recruited for participation into studies, because pet owners usually have a close and trusting relationship with their primary care veterinarian. Benefits for participating practitioners include intellectual challenge and expanded interaction with colleagues, a decreased sense of isolation and increased sense of connection with other practitioners, avoidance of "burn-out," an increased sense of professional balance, and enhancement of the perception of professionalism by patients [28]. Through activity in your local veterinary societies and specialty groups, you may discover that you are able to join in this type of collaborative research for the betterment of your patients and veterinary medicine.

SURVEILLANCE

In the process of capturing clinical outcomes by means of computerized records, an added functionality is created, that of a system for surveillance of disease that is veterinary based and zoonotic in origin. Because of the intimate relationship of pets in a family, companion animals can serve as excellent sentinels for human infection. Rapid and easily accessible return of information and results is important for the success of any surveillance system. In 1984, the Centers for Disease Control and Prevention initiated a program to capture data from health departments electronically, resulting in morbidity and mortality weekly reports (MMWRs) that take days rather than months to publish [29]. As a result of the national database that exists in PetWare, the Banfield record system has served as the foundation for the development of a model for syndromic surveillance, with funding provided by the Centers for Disease Control and Prevention [30]. If this type of surveillance interests you, you should become familiar with the MMWRs and institute practices in your hospital that would allow review of your data from clinical encounters to be evaluated.

SUMMARY

The veterinarian's ability to summarize and record relevant information from each pet encounter enables outcomes analysis and the transformation of clinical data into medical knowledge. The ability to do this requires multiple integrated processes, such as computerized records, standardized nomenclature, practice standards and protocols, case reviews, and analysis. Every practitioner can strive to use some or all of these processes, as discussed in this article. It all starts with a clear and complete medical record. The next step is to standardize terminology and processes (diagnostic and treatment). Finally, critical review of these outcomes is undertaken at an individual doctor level or in conjunction with other practices. The payoffs are enormous for the veterinarian, the patients, the pet families, and the profession. With this knowledge, our ability to provide the best veterinary care continues to evolve. Because the human-pet bond continues to be essential for human physiologic and psychologic health [31,32], it is incumbent on the veterinary profession to strive to support these important relationships with our pet companions by optimizing patient care.

References

[1] Kvart C, Häggström J, Pedersen HD, et al. Efficacy of enalapril for prevention of congestive heart failure in dogs with myxomatous valve disease and asymptomatic mitral regurgitation. J Vet Intern Med 2002;16(1):80–8.

[2] Grauer GF, Greco DS, Getzy DM, et al. Effects of enalapril versus placebo as a treatment for canine idiopathic glomerulonephritis. J Vet Intern Med 2000;14(5):526–33.

[3] Staff M. The CIDC Outreach Programme. University of Cambridge Web site. Accessed July 13, 2006.

[4] What is the Cochrane Collaboration? The Cochrane Collaboration Web site. Accessed July 13, 2006.

[5] Daily InfoPOEMs. InfoPOEMs Web site. Accessed July 13, 2006.

[6] British Veterinary Association. News & reports. Seeking the truth: the evidence-based approach to veterinary medicine. Vet Rec 2005;156(17):528–30.

[7] Hosgood G, Scholl DT. Evaluation of age and American Society of Anesthesiologists (ASA) physical status as risk factors for perianesthetic morbidity and mortality in the cat. J Vet Emerg Crit Care 2002;12:9–15.

[8] Brown SA, Crowell WA, Barsanti JA, et al. Beneficial effects of dietary mineral restriction in dogs with marked reduction of functional renal mass. J Am Soc Nephrol 1991;1:1169–79.

[9] Solomon JL, Dechter M. Are patients pleased with computer use in the examination room? J Fam Pract 1995;41:241–4.

[10] Veterinary Medical Database Web site. Accessed July 13, 2006.

[11] Lund EM, Armstrong PJ, Kirk CA, et al. Health status and population characteristics of dogs and cats examined at private veterinary practices in the United States. J Am Vet Med Assoc 1999;214:1336–41.

[12] Bishop CW, Ewing P. Representing medical knowledge: reconciling the present of creating the future? MD Comput 1992;9(4):218–25.

[13] Chisholm J. The Read clinical classification [editorial] [see comments]. Br Med J 1990;300: 1092.

[14] Lund EM, Klausner JS, Ellis LB, et al. PetTerms: a standardized nomenclature for companion animal practice. Online J Vet Res 1998;2:64–86. Available at: http://www.cpb.ouhsc.edu/ojvr/htm/. Accessed July 10, 2006.

[15] Unified Medical Language System (UMLS) Web site. Accessed July 13, 2006.

[16] Fonarow GC. Hospital protocols and evidence-based therapies: the importance of integrating aldosterone blockade into the management of patients with post-acute myocardial infarction heart failure. Clin Cardiol 2006;29(1):4–8.

[17] Becker K, Semrow S. Standardizing the care of detox patients to achieve quality outcomes. J Psychosoc Nurs Ment Health Serv 2006;44(3):33–8.

[18] Skupski DW, Lowenwirt IP, Weinbaum FI, et al. Improving hospital systems for the care of women with major obstetric hemorrhage. Obstet Gynecol 2006;107(5):977–83.

[19] Bahtsevani C, Uden G, Willman A. Outcomes of evidence-based clinical practice guidelines: a systematic review. Int J Technol Assess Health Care 2004;20(4):427–33.

[20] Epstein RS, Sherwood LM. From outcomes research to disease management: a guide for the perplexed [see comments]. Ann Intern Med 1996;124:832–7.

[21] DataSavant. Internal report: FeLV and FIV data report. DS05007. 2006 Feb.

[22] Moore GE, Guptill LF, Ward MP, et al. Adverse events diagnosed within three days of vaccine administration in dogs. J Am Vet Med Assoc 2005;227:1102–8.

[23] De Santis AC, Raghavan M, Caldanaro RJ, et al. Estimated prevalence of nematode parasitism among pet cats in the United States. J Am Vet Med Assoc 2006;228(6):885–92.

[24] Glickman LT, Glickman NW, Moore GE, et al. The safety profile of ProHeart 6 (moxidectin) and two oral heartworm preventives in dogs. Intern J Appl Res Vet Med 2005;3:49–61.

[25] Green LA, Hames CG Sr, Nutting PA. Potential of practice-based research networks: experiences from ASPN. Ambulatory Sentinel Practice Network. J Fam Pract 1994;38:400–6.

[26] Neaton J. Relative efficiency of taking research to the patient. Presented at the 13th Annual Meeting for Society for Clinical Trials, Philadelphia, PA, May 1992.

[27] Christoffel KK, Binns HJ, Stockman JA, et al. Practice-based research: opportunities and obstacles. Pediatrics 1988;82:399–406.

[28] Niebauer L, Nutting PA. Practice-based research networks: the view from the office. J Fam Pract 1994;38:409 14.

[29] Graitcer PL, Burton AH. The Epidemiologic Surveillance Project: a computer-based system for disease surveillance. Am J Prev Med 1987;3:123–7.

[30] Glickman LT, Moore GE, Glickman NW, et al. Purdue University-Banfield National Companion Animal Surveillance Program for emerging and zoonotic diseases. Vector-Borne Zoonotic Dis 2006;6:12–23.

[31] Jorgenson J. Therapeutic use of companion animals in health care. J Nurs Sch 1997;29(3):249–54.

[32] Bustad LK. Reflections on the human-animal bond. J Am Vet Med Assoc 1996;208(2):203–5.

Vet Clin Small Anim 37 (2007) 533–558

VETERINARY CLINICS
SMALL ANIMAL PRACTICE

EVIER
NDERS

Evidence-Based Management of Feline Lower Urinary Tract Disease

S. Dru Forrester, DVM, MS*, Philip Roudebush, DVM

Scientific Affairs, Hill's Pet Nutrition, 400 SW 8th Avenue, Topeka, KS 66603, USA

Feline lower urinary tract disease (FLUTD) includes any disorder affecting the urinary bladder or urethra of cats (eg, uroliths, urethral plugs, bacterial infection). Regardless of the underlying cause, FLUTD is most often associated with clinical signs that include hematuria, stranguria, dysuria, pollakiuria, and periuria (ie, urinating in inappropriate places outside or around the litter box). Diagnostic evaluation consisting of urinalysis, diagnostic imaging (abdominal radiographs or ultrasound and cystourethrography), and urine culture is needed to identify the underlying cause. If no cause is found after thorough evaluation, a diagnosis of feline idiopathic cystitis (FIC) is made.

FLUTD has been reported in 4.6% of cats evaluated in private practices in the United States and in 7% to 8% of cats evaluated at veterinary teaching hospitals [1–4]. It most often occurs in cats between the ages of 1 and 10 years [1]. The most common cause of lower urinary tract signs in cats less than 10 years of age is FIC (55%–64%); other causes include urolithiasis (15%–21%), urethral plugs (10%–21%), anatomic defects (10%), behavioral disorders (9%), neoplasia (1%–2%), and urinary tract infection (UTI; 1%–8%) [4–6]. The occurrence of UTI varies depending on the geographic location, age of the cat, and presence of concomitant disorders. In the United States, only 1% to 3% of cats with FLUTD have UTI, whereas 22% of cats with FLUTD in a Norwegian study and 8% of cats with FLUTD in a study in Switzerland had UTI [3–7]. UTI is more common in older cats (approximately 50% of cats >10 years of age had UTI in one study) and those with chronic kidney disease (10%–50% have UTI) or in cats that have had urinary tract procedures (eg, urethral catheterization, perineal urethrostomy) performed [1,8–11].

Over the past 25 years in North America, the prevalence of urolith types has changed in cats. In 1981, 78% of feline uroliths analyzed at the Minnesota Urolith Center were struvite and only 2% were calcium oxalate [12]. During the period from 1994 to 2002, the occurrence of calcium oxalate uroliths increased to 55% and that of struvite uroliths decreased to 33%. Since 2001, however, the number of struvite uroliths has gradually increased, whereas the occurrence

*Corresponding author. E-mail address: dru_forrester@hillspet.com (S.D. Forrester).

of calcium oxalate uroliths has decreased (Fig. 1). In 2006, 50% of feline uro-liths analyzed at the Minnesota Urolith Center were struvite and 39% were cal-cium oxalate (Carl A. Osborne, personal communication, 2007). A similar trend was recently reported from the Urinary Stone Analysis Laboratory at the University of California, Davis, wherein 44% of feline uroliths submitted from 2002 to 2004 were struvite and 40% were calcium oxalate [13].

Although these data are helpful, they cannot be used to determine the inci-dence (ie, rate of occurrence of new cases in the population) or prevalence (ie, total number of urolith cases during a given period) of urolith types for several reasons. Not all cats with uroliths are diagnosed (eg, they may not receive vet-erinary care) or treated (eg, their owner may decide not to treat). In addition, not all uroliths are submitted to commercial laboratories or academic centers for quantitative analysis. Finally, some urolith types are more likely to be submitted for evaluation than others. For example, if struvite uroliths are suspected, medical dissolution may be used effectively to eliminate uroliths. In contrast, if calcium oxalate uroliths are suspected, they are more likely to be removed and submitted for quantitative analysis. This would result in an underestimation of the occurrence of struvite uroliths and an overestimation of the occurrence of calcium oxalate uroliths.

In contrast to uroliths, most urethral plugs in cats are composed of struvite; this has been a consistent finding for the past 25 years. Of plugs submitted for quantitative analysis in Canada and the United States in the past 5 to 7 years, 81% to 87% were composed of struvite; less than 1% of plugs were composed of calcium oxalate [12,14].

APPLICATION OF EVIDENCE-BASED MEDICINE

Evidence-based medicine is the integration of the best research evidence and clinical expertise with consideration of patient, guardian, and owner preferences [15–18]. Veterinarians making therapeutic decisions should consider the quality of evidence supporting a recommendation to use (or not use) a particular

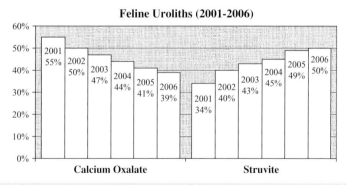

Fig. 1. Occurrence of calcium oxalate and struvite uroliths analyzed at the Minnesota Urolith Center from 2001 to 2006. During this 6-year period, there has been a gradual decline in calcium oxalate uroliths with a concomitant increase in struvite uroliths.

treatment. Whenever possible, recommendations should be based on results of randomized and controlled scientific studies (ie, the highest quality of evidence), because this is the best predictor of results likely to occur in clinical patients. In the absence of such studies, however, one should recognize inherent limitations of recommendations based on less secure forms of evidence. For dealing with such limitations, one suggested method is to assign a score defining the strength and quality of evidence (Table 1) [16]. Grade I and II evidence is highest in quality, whereas grade IV would be evidence with the lowest quality. Such a scoring system recognizes that the quality of evidence supporting a recommendation is an important consideration when making therapeutic decisions.

Although recommendations have been made for treating patients with FLUTD, only a few have been carefully studied in cats with naturally occurring disease. This article reviews evidence that supports currently recommended treatments for the most common causes of FLUTD in cats: FIC, struvite uroliths and urethral plugs, and calcium oxalate uroliths.

FELINE IDIOPATHIC CYSTITIS

FIC is characterized by relapses of lower urinary tract signs (hematuria, pollakiuria, stranguria, and periuria) that often resolve spontaneously within 4 to 7 days with or without treatment. This condition has been called many names, including feline urologic syndrome, idiopathic FLUTD, and interstitial cystitis. Throughout this article, the acronym FIC is used. Although our understanding of the pathogenesis of FIC has improved over the past decade, the underlying cause remains unknown. Therefore, reasonable goals of managing cats with FIC are to decrease the severity of clinical signs and to increase the interval

Table 1
Descriptions of grades used to classify evidence

Grade	Description of evidence
I	At least one properly designed randomized controlled clinical study performed in patients of the target species
II	Evidence from properly designed randomized controlled studies in animals of the target species with spontaneous disease in a laboratory or research animal colony setting
III	Appropriately controlled studies without randomization Appropriately designed case-control epidemiologic studies Studies using models of disease or simulations in the target species Dramatic results from uncontrolled studies Case series
IV	Studies conducted in other species Reports of expert committees Descriptive studies Case reports Pathophysiologic justification/rationale Opinions of respected experts

From Roudebush P, Allen TA, Dodd CE, et al. Application of evidence-based medicine to veterinary clinical nutrition. J Am Vet Med Assoc 2004;224:1768; with permission.

between episodes of FLUTD [19]. This can be facilitated by educating owners of cats about known factors involved in the pathogenesis of FIC and working closely with them to establish a therapeutic regimen that is best for their cat.

Over the past 40 years, numerous treatments have been recommended to control signs in cats with FIC; however, only a few have been evaluated in clinical trials of cats with FIC [20]. The currently recommended standard of care for cats with FIC includes environmental enrichment, stress reduction, feeding moist food (>60% moisture), and using additional strategies to increase water intake [21,22]. Additional treatments (eg, analgesics) may help to minimize clinical signs and pain during acute episodes. For cats with severe recurrent episodes of FIC, administration of such agents as glycosaminoglycans (GAGs) and amitriptyline may be considered in addition to standard treatment.

Environmental Enrichment and Stress Reduction

In cats with FIC, there seems to be an imbalance in the neuroendocrine system, such that excitatory sympathetic nervous system outflow is inadequately controlled by cortisol [21]. This increased activity may cause increased tissue permeability of the urinary bladder, resulting in increased sensory afferent activity and clinical signs of FIC. Because of these abnormalities, treatment aimed at decreasing central noradrenergic drive (eg, stress) may be important for managing cats with FIC.

Environmental enrichment and stress reduction are recommended as part of the initial management of cats with FIC [21,22]. Environmental enrichment is the process of improving or enhancing an animal's environment and care within the context of its behavioral biology and natural history; the goal is to increase behavioral choices and draw out species-appropriate behaviors [23]. For indoor-housed cats with FIC, this has been defined as providing all necessary resources, enhancing interactions with owners, minimizing conflict, and making any changes gradually [21]. Some components of environmental enrichment include providing opportunities for play and resting (eg, horizontal and vertical surfaces for scratching, hiding places, climbing platforms) and a quiet location for cats to eat alone. Litter box care and maintenance also play an important role. More detailed information on environmental enrichment is available elsewhere [19,24,25].

Although environmental enrichment has been recommended for cats with FIC and is believed to be beneficial, it has not been evaluated in randomized controlled clinical trials. Recently, a prospective observational study evaluating the effects of multimodal environmental modification was reported in 46 client-owned cats with FIC [26]. There were significant reductions in lower urinary tract signs, fearfulness, and nervousness after treatment for 10 months. Based on these findings, randomized controlled clinical studies evaluating the effectiveness of environmental enrichment in cats with FIC were recommended [26].

Recommendations
- Institute environmental enrichment and methods to reduce stress as part of the initial management of all cats with FIC.

- Consult additional resources with helpful information that can be used by veterinarians and cat owners [19,24,25].

Evidence

The best evidence supporting these recommendations comes from a prospective clinical study in cats with FIC, pathophysiologic rationale, clinical experiences, and expert opinion (grade III).

Nutritional Management
Moist food

Nutritional management of cats with FIC (ie, methods to increase water intake) has been recommended to dilute urine, which may decrease the concentration of substances in urine that are irritating to the urinary bladder mucosa. Feeding moist food has been associated with an increase in daily water intake and urine volume in cats compared with feeding dry food. Although healthy cats drink more water when eating dry food compared with moist food, the total volume of water ingested (ie, drinking water plus water in food) is significantly greater when cats are fed moist food and more water is excreted in urine versus feces [27,28]. Feeding frequency also seems to affect water intake in cats. In a study of healthy adult cats, water intake (in addition to that consumed in the food) increased significantly when cats were fed two or three meals compared with a single meal each day [29].

In a 1-year nonrandomized prospective study of 46 cats with FIC, feeding a moist therapeutic food (Royal Canin Veterinary Diet feline Urinary SO in Gel [St. Charles, Missouri]) was associated with significant improvement compared with feeding a dry version of the same food [30]. At the end of the 1-year study, recurrence of clinical signs in cats eating moist food was significantly less (11% of 18 cats) compared with cats eating dry food (39% of 28 cats) ($P = .04$) [30]. Compared with the dry food group, urine specific gravity was significantly less in cats eating moist food; throughout the 1-year study, mean urine specific gravity values ranged from 1.032 to 1.041 in cats eating moist food and from 1.051 to 1.052 in cats eating dry food ($P < .05$).

In a study evaluating glucosamine in cats with FIC (see section on GAGs), most cats in both groups (glucosamine and placebo) improved significantly compared with their condition at the beginning of the study. Initially, 38 cats (95%) were fed dry food exclusively, or at least half of their food was in dry form. Owners were given client education handouts describing management of cats with FIC, including feeding moist food. After starting the clinical study, 36 (90%) owners increased the amount of moist food given to their cats, such that at least 50% of their cats' daily intake was moist food. In 33 cats (82.5%), owners began feeding moist food exclusively. Mean urine specific gravity at the beginning of the study was 1.050 ± 1.007; this value was significantly lower (1.036 ± 1.010) when reassessed 1 month later ($P < .01$). The change in urine specific gravity coincided with the change in food formulation and initial improvement in mean monthly clinical scores. It is likely that increased consumption of moist food caused the urine dilution, which, in turn, was associated with improved health scores. It is also possible that other factors associated with feeding moist food (eg, texture, taste, owner-cat interactions associated with delivery of moist food) played a role, however.

Recommendations.
- Recommend gradual transition to moist food when FIC is diagnosed. For some cats, this transition may require weeks to months to implement. More detailed information on feeding cats with FIC is available elsewhere [21,22,24].
- Try to maintain urine specific gravity values less than 1.040 or lower based on clinical signs. Measure urine specific gravity using a refractometer, which is more accurate than urine dipsticks [31].
- Consider feeding two to three meals per day instead of a single meal.

Evidence. The best evidence supporting these recommendations comes from a clinical study of cats with FIC being fed the moist version of one therapeutic food (Royal Canin Veterinary Diet feline Urinary SO), a clinical study of cats with FIC being fed moist foods, and studies in healthy cats as well as pathophysiologic rationale, expert opinion, and clinical experience (grade III).

Increased salt intake
Increasing the sodium chloride content of food (1.0%–1.4% sodium, dry matter basis [DMB]) has been used as a method to increase water intake and urine volume and to cause subsequent urine dilution [32–36]. It is generally believed that urine dilution is helpful because it may dilute substances that are potentially irritating to the urinary bladder mucosa. Use of increased dietary salt alone has not been compared with other methods to stimulate urine dilution in cats with FIC.

At present, there are differing opinions regarding the safety of feeding high-sodium foods to cats [35,37,38]. According to the most recent information published by the National Research Council (NRC), it is difficult to suggest a safe upper limit of sodium for healthy adult cats [39]. The NRC has concluded that as long as unlimited amounts of water are available, it is likely that cats can tolerate reasonably high concentrations of dietary sodium; the safe upper limit of sodium for adult cats has been defined as 1.5% sodium (DMB) [39]. The safe upper limit of sodium for cats with chronic kidney disease, FLUTD, and other conditions is unknown, however.

Long-term consequences of high-sodium foods have not been evaluated in healthy cats or in cats with hypertension, and the effect of sodium on kidney function remains controversial [35,37,40,41]. Based on information currently available, feeding high-sodium foods has not been associated with hypertension in healthy cats or in cats with kidney disease (naturally occurring or experimentally induced) [34,35,40]. These studies were designed to evaluate cats for periods ranging from 7 days to 3 months; therefore, effects beyond this time frame are unknown. In a case-control study of 38 cats with chronic kidney disease diagnosed during a 1-year period (1994–1995), pet owners were interviewed about the foods their cat received in the 3 years before diagnosis of kidney disease

[41]. Results revealed an association between increased dietary sodium and decreased odds of kidney disease; however, because of the nature of epidemiologic studies, additional evaluation is necessary to show a cause-and-effect relation. In another study, cats with an experimentally induced model of kidney disease were fed different levels of sodium for 7 days; feeding the lowest amount of sodium chloride was associated with urinary potassium loss and reduced glomerular filtration [40]. The authors concluded that low sodium intake might contribute to progressive renal injury in cats. In a 2-year study, cats with naturally occurring kidney disease lived significantly longer and had no uremic episodes when fed a renal therapeutic food with a similar amount of sodium as that used in the previous study versus a control food (with higher sodium) [42]. Finally, the effects of high-salt intake (1.2% sodium, DMB) for 3 months were evaluated in cats with mild azotemia attributable to naturally occurring chronic kidney disease [35]. These cats had progressive increases in blood urea nitrogen (BUN), serum creatinine, and serum phosphorus compared with cats consuming food with 0.4% sodium (DMB). Based on all findings to date, it seems that further study is needed to determine better the role of sodium in healthy cats fed long term as well as in cats with hypertension and chronic kidney disease.

Recommendations.
- Consider using high-salt foods in cats with FIC if clinical signs continue after implementing environmental enrichment, stress reduction, and feeding moist food.
- Do not use high-salt foods in cats with kidney disease.
- Monitor kidney function and blood pressure in cats at risk for kidney disease or hypertension when feeding high-salt foods.

Evidence. The best evidence supporting these recommendations comes from pathophysiologic rationale, studies in healthy cats, and studies in cats with naturally occurring kidney disease (grade IV [for using high-salt foods in cats with FIC]).

Other methods to increase water intake
Additional methods to increase water intake in cats with FIC include adding broth or water to food and using water fountains, special water bowls, or running faucets. At present, none of these treatments has been evaluated in cats with FIC.

Recommendations.
- Consider using additional methods to increase water intake if cats do not eat moist food or if clinical signs continue after beginning treatment with moist food.

Evidence. The best evidence supporting these recommendations comes from pathophysiologic rationale and expert opinion (grade IV).

Amitriptyline
Amitriptyline (Elavil; AstraZeneca Pharmaceuticals, Wilmington, Delaware) is a tricycle antidepressant with anticholinergic, antihistaminic, sympatholytic,

analgesic, and anti-inflammatory properties that has been used in cats with FIC and in women with interstitial cystitis (a condition similar to FIC) [43–46]. In an uncontrolled study of cats with severe recurrent FIC that failed to respond to other treatments, administration of amitriptyline for 12 months was associated with decreased clinical signs in 9 (60%) of 15 cats during the last 6 months of treatment [43]. A randomized controlled clinical trial of amitriptyline treatment for 7 days revealed no significant difference in the rate of recovery from pollakiuria or hematuria; overall, clinical signs recurred significantly faster and more frequently in cats treated with amitriptyline compared with control cats [44]. In a similar study, amitriptyline combined with amoxicillin was no more effective than placebo and amoxicillin when given for 7 days to cats with FIC [45]. Based on current information, amitriptyline does not seem to be beneficial for short-term management of cats with FIC. It is possible that longer use (minimum of weeks to months) may be helpful, however.

Recommendations

- There is insufficient evidence to recommend short-term (ie, 7 days) treatment with amitriptyline.
- Consider long-term treatment with amitriptyline (5–10 mg per cat administered by mouth once daily) when cats with FIC continue to have severe or recurrent episodes despite increased water intake and use of environmental enrichment and stress reduction.

Evidence

The best evidence supporting these recommendations comes from two clinical studies of cats with FIC in which treatment with amitriptyline for 7 days was not effective compared with placebo [44,45]. In another prospective clinical study, amitriptyline seemed to be beneficial when cats were treated for 6 to 12 months [43] (grade III [for long-term treatment]).

Anti-Inflammatory Agents and Analgesics

These agents have been recommended to help manage discomfort in cats with FIC, especially during acute episodes. There have been no clinical trials evaluating opioid analgesics (eg, butorphanol) or nonsteroidal anti-inflammatory drugs (eg, meloxicam, piroxicam) in cats with FIC. Prednisolone (1 mg/kg administered by mouth twice daily for 10 days) was evaluated in a double-blind randomized controlled clinical trial of 12 cats with FIC and was found to be no more effective than placebo for reducing the severity or duration of clinical signs in affected cats [47].

Recommendations

- Consider using analgesics and anti-inflammatory agents to help manage patient discomfort during acute episodes of FIC.
- Drugs that may be used 3–4 days for initial pain management include butorphanol (0.4 mg/kg administered by mouth every 8 hours) and meloxicam (0.1 mg/kg administered by mouth once daily).
- Other analgesics and anti-inflammatory agents may be appropriate; selection is often based on clinician preference or experience.

- There is insufficient evidence to recommend the use of prednisolone for cats with FIC.

Evidence
The best evidence supporting the use of analgesics and nonsteroidal anti-inflammatory agents comes from expert opinion and pathophysiologic rationale (grade IV [for analgesics and nonsteroidal anti-inflammatory agents]).

Feline Facial Pheromone

Synthetic feline facial pheromone therapy has been recommended to decrease signs of stress in cats with FIC. In a double-blind placebo-controlled clinical study of 20 hospitalized cats (13 with FLUTD and 7 apparently healthy), exposure to feline facial pheromone (Feliway; Veterinary Products Laboratories, Phoenix, Arizona) was associated with significant increases in grooming, interest in food, and food intake; these results suggested that feline facial pheromone had an anxiolytic effect in some cats [48]. Feline facial pheromone (Feliway; Ceva Animal Health, Libourne, France) also was evaluated in a small study of 12 cats with FIC [49]. Although there was no significant difference between treatment of the environment with placebo and feline facial pheromone for 2 months, there was a trend for cats exposed to facial pheromone to show fewer days with clinical signs of cystitis, a reduced number of episodes, and reduced negative behavioral traits (less aggression and fear). Because of the small number of patients evaluated and the trend for improvement in cats exposed to facial pheromone, additional evaluation of a larger number of cats is warranted.

Recommendations
- Consider treatment with feline facial pheromones in cats with signs of stress or when clinical signs persist after implementing environmental enrichment and methods to increase water intake.

Evidence
The best evidence supporting these recommendations comes from prospective clinical studies, pathophysiologic rationale, clinical experience, and expert opinion (grade III/IV).

Glycosaminoglycans

Treatment with GAGs (eg, pentosan polysulfate, glucosamine, chondroitin sulfate) has been suggested in cats with FIC, because defects in the GAG layer covering the urinary bladder epithelium may play a role in the pathogenesis of the disease. These agents seem to be useful in women with interstitial cystitis, a condition similar to FIC [46,50,51]. A randomized, double-blind, placebo-controlled study was conducted to determine whether administration of glucosamine (Cystease, 125 mg administered per mouth once daily for 6 months; Ceva Animal Health) would reduce the severity or recurrence rate of clinical signs in cats with FIC compared with placebo [52]. Owner assessments suggested that glucosamine-treated cats achieved a slightly greater improvement by the end of the study (mean health score: 4.4 ± 0.7) compared with the placebo group (mean health score: 3.9 ± 1.6); however, this difference was not statistically significant ($P > .05$).

Recommendations
- Consider using GAGs in cats that have continued clinical signs after implementation of environmental enrichment, stress reduction, and methods to increase water intake.
- Agents that have been recommended include pentosan polysulfate (Elmiron, 8 mg/kg administered by mouth every 12 hours; Ortho-McNeil Pharmaceutical, Raritan, New Jersey) and a combination of glucosamine/chondroitin sulfate (Cosequin, 125 mg/100 mg per 4.5 kg cat administered by mouth every 24 hours; Nutramax Laboratories, Edgewood, Maryland).
- There is insufficient evidence to support use of glucosamine alone at this time.

Evidence
The best evidence supporting the use of GAGs comes from human studies, pathophysiologic rationale, expert opinions, and clinical experience. Because of possible synergy between glucosamine and chondroitin sulfate, additional study of this combination is indicated [20] (grade IV [for GAGs like pentosan polysulfate or a combination of glucosamine and chondroitin sulfate]).

Fluid Therapy

Administration of subcutaneous fluids was evaluated in a study of cats with FIC [53]. At the beginning of the study, cats were randomly assigned to receive no treatment (10 cats) or lactated Ringer's solution (100 mL) once (9 cats). Five days later, owners were contacted regarding response to treatment. Among cats that received fluid therapy, 7 had a complete response and 2 had a partial response. Of cats that received no treatment, 7 had a complete response, 1 had a partial response, and 2 had no response. There was no significant difference in responses when the two groups were compared.

Recommendations
- There is insufficient evidence to support one-time treatment with lactated Ringer's solution for cats with FIC.

Evidence
The best evidence supporting these findings comes from a clinical study in cats with FIC (grade I [single treatment with lactated Ringer's solution is not effective]).

Propantheline

Propantheline (Pro-Banthine; Searle, Skokie, Illinois), an anticholinergic drug that causes urinary bladder relaxation, has been recommended for treatment of cats with urge incontinence associated with FIC. This drug was evaluated in a small study of cats with FIC; there was no significant difference in resolution of clinical signs in cats receiving a single dose of propantheline (7.5 mg administered by mouth) compared with no treatment [53].

Recommendations
- There is insufficient evidence to support using a single dose of propantheline for cats with FIC.
- If there is no response to analgesics or nonsteroidal anti-inflammatory drugs during acute episodes of FIC, consider different dosage regimens of propantheline (0.25–0.5 mg/kg administered by mouth every 12–24 hours).

Evidence
The best evidence supporting these recommendations comes from pathophysiologic rationale and a clinical study in cats with FIC (grades I [single dose is not effective] and IV [for use of other dosage regimens]).

Antimicrobials

Antimicrobials have long been recommended and used in cats with FIC, probably because they seem to be associated with resolution of clinical signs and many veterinarians feel the need to offer some treatment to frustrated owners of cats with FIC. In a study of cats with FIC, resolution of clinical signs was not significantly different when cats were treated three times daily with chloramphenicol versus placebo [53]. Based on the rare occurrence of UTI in most middle-aged cats with FLUTD, antimicrobial treatment is rarely indicated.

Recommendations
- There is insufficient evidence to recommend routine use of antimicrobials in cats with FIC.
- Begin appropriate antimicrobial treatment if UTI is diagnosed by urine culture in a cat with signs of FLUTD.

Evidence
The best evidence supporting these recommendations comes from a small randomized controlled clinical study in cats with FIC, pathophysiologic rationale, and expert opinions (grades I and IV [that routine antimicrobial treatment is not indicated]).

TREATMENT OF STRUVITE UROLITHIASIS

Treatment of cats with struvite uroliths includes physical removal of uroliths (eg, cystotomy, voiding urohydropropulsion, laser lithotripsy) or dissolution by means of nutritional management. There have been no studies comparing these methods of treatment with each other. The choice of treatment method depends on clinician experience and expertise, availability of special equipment, patient factors, and client preferences. Several therapeutic foods marketed for dissolution of struvite uroliths are formulated to avoid excessive magnesium and phosphorus and to maintain acidic urine pH; this decreases precursors available to form uroliths and increases struvite solubility in urine. Some foods contain relatively high amounts of salt (eg, sodium chloride), which results in production of more dilute urine and decreased saturation of struvite in urine (Table 2).

Table 2
Nutrient information for commercially available foods for cats with feline lower urinary tract disease[a]

Company	Food	Form	Indications	Na	Mg	Ca	P	n-3	Target urine pH
Hill's	Prescription Diet c/d Multicare Feline	Moist	SP, C, FIC	0.32	0.052	0.72	0.68	0.96	6.2–6.4
Hill's	Prescription Diet c/d Multicare Feline	Dry	SP, C, FIC	0.33	0.061	0.76	0.65	0.64	6.2–6.4
Hill's	Prescription Diet s/d Feline	Moist	SD	0.41	0.062	0.62	0.48	0.34	5.9–6.1
Hill's	Prescription Diet s/d Feline	Dry	SD	0.40	0.059	1.05	0.77	0.26	5.9–6.1
Hill's	Prescription Diet x/d with Chicken Feline	Moist	C/FIC	0.37	0.082	0.69	0.53	0.15	6.6–6.8
Hill's	Prescription Diet x/d Feline	Dry	C	0.36	0.076	0.76	0.66	0.16	6.6–6.8
Hill's	Prescription Diet w/d Feline	Moist	SP/C/FIC	0.33	0.063	0.74	0.59	0.15	6.2–6.4
Hill's	Prescription Diet w/d Feline	Dry	SP/C	0.30	0.059	0.99	0.77	0.25	6.2–6.4
Iams	Low pH/S/Feline Formula	Moist	SP/FIC	0.46	0.1	1.27	1.0	NA	5.9–6.3
Iams	Low pH/S/Feline Formula	Dry	SP	0.52	0.084	1.10	0.96	0.40	5.9–6.3
Iams	Moderate pH/O/Feline Formula	Moist	C/FIC	0.48	0.104	1.23	0.90	NA	6.3–6.9
Iams	Moderate pH/O/Feline Formula	Dry	C	0.48	0.088	1.11	0.96	NA	6.3–6.9
Purina	ONE Special Care Urinary Tract Health Formula	Dry	SP	0.2	0.07	1.09	0.99	NA	<6.3
Purina	Pro Plan Urinary Tract Health Formula Extra Care	Dry	SP	0.26	0.070	1.05	1.01	NA	6.2–6.4

Manufacturer	Product	Form	Indication						pH
Purina	UR URinary St/Ox Feline Formula	Moist	SD/SP/C/FIC	0.62	0.07	0.96	0.97	NA	6.0–6.4
Purina	UR URinary St/Ox Feline Formula	Soft/Moist	SP/C	0.28	0.12	1.64	1.78	NA	6.0–6.4
Purina	UR URinary St/Ox Feline Formula	Dry	SD/SP/C	1.17	0.07	1.10	1.08	NA	6.0–6.4
Royal Canin	Veterinary Diet Control Formula	Moist	SP/FIC	0.44	0.08	1.12	1.00	NA	6.0–6.3
Royal Canin	Veterinary Diet Control Formula	Dry	SP	0.71	0.06	0.96	0.65	NA	6.0–6.3
Royal Canin	Medi-Cal Preventive Formula	Moist	SP/FIC	0.3	0.06	1.10	1.00	NA	NA
Royal Canin	Medi-Cal Preventive Formula	Dry	SP	0.4	0.07	1.00	0.80	NA	NA
Royal Canin	Medi-Cal Dissolution Formula	Moist	SD	1.27	NA	1.08	1.06	NA	NA
Royal Canin	Medi-Cal Dissolution Formula	Dry	SD	0.37	NA	0.97	0.97	NA	NA
Royal Canin	Veterinary Diet feline Urinary SO in Gel	Moist	SD/SP/C/FIC	1.02	0.097	1.02	1.36	NA	6.0–6.3
Royal Canin	Veterinary Diet feline Urinary SO 30	Dry	SD/SP/C	1.40	0.075	1.08	0.86	NA	6.0–6.3

Abbreviations: C, calcium oxalate; Ca, calcium; Mg, magnesium; n-3, omega-3 fatty acids; Na, sodium; NA, not available; P, phosphorus; SD, struvite dissolution; SP, struvite prevention.

ªAll nutrients are expressed on a dry matter basis.

Only two foods have been evaluated in cats with struvite uroliths. In a prospective study of cats, feeding a calculolytic food (Hill's Prescription Diet s/d Feline, Hill's Pet Nutrition, Topeka, Kansas) was associated with dissolution of sterile struvite uroliths within a mean of 36 days; cats with concurrent UTI required treatment for longer periods (2.6 months) [54]. In another prospective study, the effectiveness of moist and dry versions of a calculolytic food (Medi-Cal/Royal Canin Feline Dissolution Formula, Veterinary Medical Diets, Guelph, Ontario, Canada) was evaluated in cats with suspected or confirmed struvite uroliths [55]. The average time to urolith dissolution in both groups (moist and dry food) was 4.28 weeks.

In addition to clinical studies in cats with struvite uroliths, there have been reports describing use of surrogate markers, such as relative supersaturation (RSS) and activity product ratio (APR) in healthy cats to identify the risk for struvite urolith formation [56–59]. These measurements are used to estimate saturation of urine with several stone-forming minerals; decreased values indicate a lower risk for crystalluria and urolith formation. It has been reported that struvite RSS values less than 1 indicate that urine is undersaturated with struvite and that struvite crystals do not form but dissolve [37,58]. Several studies have measured struvite RSS values in healthy cats fed different foods and have found values less than 1 [56,60–63]. The authors are unaware of any studies of RSS or APR values in cats with struvite uroliths or studies correlating these values with recurrence of uroliths in cats with struvite disease.

Recommendations

- For cats with suspected struvite uroliths (usually cats <7 years old, alkaline urine pH, struvite crystalluria, or radiopaque uroliths), transition to feeding a canned calculolytic food (Medi-Cal/Royal Canin Feline Dissolution Formula or Hill's Prescription Diet s/d Feline) over a 7-day period.
- Re-evaluate cats every 2 to 4 weeks by performing urinalysis and abdominal radiographs. Urine pH should remain acidic, and specific gravity should be less than 1.040 if canned food is being fed exclusively. Continue nutritional management for 1 month beyond radiographic resolution of the urolith.
- If uroliths do not dissolve completely or noticeably decrease in size within 2 months, there are several options. First, if the patient is eating dry food, gradually transition to moist food only. If the patient is already being fed moist food, consider changing to a different therapeutic food marketed for struvite dissolution or using additional strategies to increase water intake. If uroliths persist despite these changes and the pet owner is adhering to nutritional recommendations, another urolith type (eg, calcium oxalate, compound urolith) is likely. Removal of uroliths and submission for quantitative analysis are indicated.
- Because of the risk for worsening kidney function, do not use high-salt foods (see Table 2) in cats with kidney disease.

Evidence

The best evidence supporting these recommendations comes from prospective clinical studies in cats with struvite uroliths, measurements of surrogate markers in healthy cats, pathophysiologic rationale, expert opinions, and clinical experience (grades III [for Hill's Prescription Diet s/d Feline and Medi-Cal/Royal Canin Feline Dissolution Formula] and IV [for other therapeutic foods formulated to dissolve struvite uroliths]).

PREVENTING RECURRENCE OF STRUVITE UROLITHS AND URETHRAL PLUGS

There are several commercial foods available for preventing recurrence of struvite uroliths and urethral plugs (see Table 2). These foods are similar to dissolution foods; however, target urine pH is generally higher in preventive foods. In a randomized prospective study of cats with urethral plugs (suspected or confirmed to be struvite), the effectiveness of feeding a calculolytic food (Hill's Prescription Diet s/d Feline) was compared with perineal urethrostomy alone and perineal urethrostomy plus the calculolytic food [11]. Transient microscopic hematuria occurred in 25% of cats in all treatment groups; however, urethral obstruction was not observed in any group during the 1-year study. This study did not include an untreated control group; however, the recurrence rate for urethral obstruction in a previous study was 35% [64]. Bacterial UTI occurred in 40% to 50% of cats that had perineal urethrostomies but was not observed in cats managed by calculolytic food alone.

Values for RSS and APR have been determined in healthy cats consuming several foods formulated for struvite prevention. In a study of healthy cats, values for struvite APR and RSS were consistent with urinary undersaturation with struvite for three dry foods (Hill's Prescription Diet c/d Feline, Hill's Prescription Diet s/d Feline, and Purina UR Urinary Feline Formula, Nestlè Purina PetCare Company, St. Louis, Missouri) [62]. In another study, RSS for struvite was significantly decreased in healthy cats fed dry formulas of Purina UR Urinary Feline Formula or Hill's Prescription Diet c/d Feline compared with other foods [56]. In a study of six healthy cats, struvite APR was lowest in cats fed Hill's Prescription Diet c/d Feline compared with other foods (Royal Canin Veterinary Cats Young Adult, Hill's Hairball Control, and Eukanuba Veterinary Diets Low pH, The Iams Company, Dayton, Ohio); however, all foods resulted in APR values less than 1 [60]. Other commercially available preventive foods (Royal Canin Veterinary Diet Feline Urinary SO moist and dry formulas and Purina UR URinary St/Ox Feline Formula moist and dry formulas) also are reported to result in production of urine with struvite RSS values less than 1 when fed to healthy cats [61,65]. Again, there are no reports describing RSS or APR values in cats with struvite disease or correlating these values with disease recurrence.

Recommendations
- After dissolution or removal of struvite uroliths, gradually transition to a food formulated to prevent struvite crystalluria and urolith formation.
- Follow guidelines established by the manufacturer of the selected food.
- Consider using a dissolution (calculolytic) food for initial management (1–3 months) after relieving urethral obstruction. Then change to a struvite preventive food formulated for maintenance needs (see Table 2).

Evidence

The best evidence supporting these recommendations comes from a prospective clinical study in cats with urethral plugs and studies evaluating effects of other foods on urinary struvite saturation in healthy cats [11,56,61,62,65] (grades III [for Hill's Prescription Diet s/d Feline in cats with urethral plugs] and IV [for other foods formulated to prevent struvite recurrence]).

CALCIUM OXALATE UROLITHIASIS

The treatment of choice for calcium oxalate urolithiasis is urolith removal, followed by methods to prevent urolith recurrence. General goals of preventive management are to decrease urine saturation with calcium oxalate, increase the concentration or activity of calcium oxalate inhibitors in urine, and promote production of urine that is more dilute. At present, the standard of care for preventing calcium oxalate urolith recurrence is to feed a moist therapeutic food and encourage water intake [22,66]. Other recommended treatments include potassium citrate, vitamin B_6, and thiazide diuretics. If hypercalcemia exists, the underlying cause should be treated; many cats have idiopathic hypercalcemia, which makes specific treatment challenging [67–69].

Although much information is available regarding risk factors for calcium oxalate uroliths, the cause remains largely unknown, making ideal preventive recommendations challenging [3,70]. In a recent epidemiologic study, cats fed foods low in sodium or potassium or formulated to maximize urine acidity had an increased risk of developing calcium oxalate uroliths, whereas foods with the highest moisture or protein contents and with moderate amounts of magnesium, phosphorus, or calcium were associated with a decreased risk of calcium oxalate uroliths [3]. The authors cautioned that the study results should not be interpreted as proof of cause-and-effect relations and adopted by pet food manufacturers; instead, the findings should be used to help design prospective studies of cats with urolithiasis. Until such information is known, treatment should be based on the quality of evidence available.

Nutritional Management

Therapeutic foods

There are several commercially available therapeutic foods for prevention of calcium oxalate uroliths in cats (see Table 2). Of these, one food (Hill's Prescription Diet x/d Feline) has been evaluated in cats with naturally occurring calcium oxalate uroliths [71]. In a study of 10 cats with confirmed calcium oxalate uroliths, urinary APR values for calcium oxalate were measured before beginning the study and after a feeding trial. Using a crossover design, half of the cats were randomly assigned to continue their regular food and the other half were fed the therapeutic food; after 8 weeks, the foods were switched and fed for another 8 weeks. Urine APR values were determined and compared between groups (ie, regular food, therapeutic food). Results revealed that hypercalciuria was a consistent abnormality in urolith-forming cats and that APR values for calcium oxalate were significantly lower in cats fed the therapeutic food compared with their regular food.

In cats with hypercalcemia and calcium oxalate uroliths, feeding increased amounts of fiber and administering potassium citrate have been recommended [66]. In a report of five cats with calcium oxalate uroliths, hypercalcemia resolved and urolith recurrence was not observed after discontinuing an acidifying food (or urinary acidifier) and changing to a higher fiber food (Hill's Prescription Diet w/d Feline) or adding a fiber supplement [69]. The duration of nutritional management and monitoring for urolith recurrence was not known for all cases. It was suggested that increased fiber may have lowered serum calcium by binding intestinal calcium, preventing its absorption or decreasing intestinal transit time through the small intestine (the area in which most calcium is absorbed).

Other foods containing relatively higher amounts of salt (> 1% sodium, DMB) have been evaluated by measuring calcium oxalate saturation in urine, primarily in healthy cats (see Table 2). Studies in healthy cats have shown that increased salt intake is associated with increased water consumption and urine dilution, which could help to prevent urolith recurrence [34,36]. Concerns have been expressed about the increasing risk for calcium oxalate uroliths attributable to increased urine calcium excretion associated with salt-induced diuresis; however, urine calcium concentration and calcium oxalate saturation were not increased in normal cats when fed a high-salt food, even though there was a significant increase in 24-hour urine calcium excretion [36]. This was likely attributable to dilution of calcium and other substances in urine associated with increased urine volume. In another study of healthy cats, increased dietary salt was associated with increased water intake and urine volume and significantly decreased values for calcium oxalate RSS [32]. Interestingly, urinary RSS for calcium oxalate was not significantly decreased when feeding high-salt foods compared with lower salt foods to healthy cats in three studies [36,60,61]. There has been a single case report describing the effects of a high-salt food (Royal Canin Feline Urinary SO) in a cat with naturally occurring calcium oxalate uroliths; calcium oxalate RSS decreased from a value around 12 to less than 1 after the cat was switched to the therapeutic food, and uroliths had not recurred for more than 2 years at the time of last evaluation [72]. To decrease the likelihood of urolith recurrence, it has been recommended that calcium oxalate RSS be maintained at less than 12, because crystalluria is more likely to develop at higher values [37]. Some therapeutic foods (Purina UR URinary St/Ox Feline Formula and Royal Canin Veterinary Diet Feline Urinary SO) have been reported to produce urine with calcium oxalate RSS values less than 5 in healthy cats [61,65]. Feeding a similar food (Royal Canin Urinary Tract Support Diet) to dogs with calcium oxalate uroliths was associated with significantly decreased calcium oxalate RSS values [73]. To date, there have been no studies evaluating RSS values and recurrence of calcium oxalate uroliths in cats.

In addition to progressive worsening of kidney function, increased fractional excretion of calcium were identified in cats (n = 6) with mild naturally occurring chronic kidney disease consuming high-salt food in one study [35]. The effects of these foods in cats with kidney disease need additional study, especially because renoliths and ureteroliths (most of which are calcium oxalate) are being diagnosed more frequently in cats with chronic kidney disease [35,74].

Recommendations.
- For initial management of cats with calcium oxalate uroliths, gradually transition to a moist therapeutic food formulated to help prevent urolith recurrence.
- For cats with hypercalcemia, treat the underlying cause if it can be found. Consider gradually transitioning to a higher fiber food and adding potassium citrate.
- The ideal treatment for calcium oxalate uroliths is unknown; therefore, all cats should be monitored for recurrence. Perform urinalysis (evaluate for calcium oxalate crystalluria) every 3 months and abdominal radiographs or ultrasound (looking for evidence of urolith recurrence) every 6 months. If uroliths recur, treatment may be changed and less invasive procedures (eg, voiding urohydropropulsion) are more likely to be effective when uroliths are smaller.

Evidence. The best evidence supporting these recommendations comes from a randomized controlled clinical study evaluating effects of one therapeutic food on calcium oxalate saturation in urine of cats with a history of calcium oxalate uroliths, effects of other therapeutic foods on calcium oxalate saturation in urine of healthy cats, case reports, results in dogs with calcium oxalate uroliths (dogs), expert opinion, and clinical experience (grades II/III [Hill's Prescription Diet x/d Feline], III/IV [high-salt foods (eg, Royal Canin Veterinary Diet feline Urinary SO, Purina UR URinary St/Ox Feline Formula)], and IV [other therapeutic foods]).

Increased water intake and moist foods
Increased water intake is associated with decreased concentrations of urolith-forming minerals in urine and has been recommended to help prevent urolith recurrence. This may be accomplished by feeding moist food, feeding more frequent meals per day, adding additional water or broth to dry or moist food, and using water fountains or novel water bowls. One epidemiologic study showed that cats fed high-moisture foods were less likely to develop calcium oxalate uroliths than cats fed low-moisture (dry) foods [75]. There have been no reported studies evaluating the effectiveness of methods to increase water intake on prevention of calcium oxalate urolith recurrence in cats.

Recommendations.
- As part of the initial management of cats with calcium oxalate uroliths, transition to moist food.
- It may also be helpful to recommend additional methods to increase water intake.
- Consider feeding two to three meals per day versus a single meal.

Evidence. The best evidence supporting these recommendations comes from an epidemiologic study of cats with calcium oxalate uroliths; pathophysiologic rationale; expert opinion; and clinical studies of healthy cats, cats with FIC, and human beings with calcium oxalate uroliths (grades III/IV [feeding moist food] and IV [multiple meals and other methods to increase water intake]).

Potassium Citrate

Potassium citrate is a urinary alkalinizer that has been recommended to prevent calcium oxalate uroliths; it is included in some therapeutic foods and may also be administered alone. In epidemiologic studies of cats, increased urine pH values (> 6.25–6.29) are associated with a lower risk of calcium oxalate uroliths [70,75]. In addition, citrate is an inhibitor of calcium oxalate; increased urinary citrate may form soluble complexes with calcium, making it unavailable to form calcium oxalate uroliths. In a study of normal dogs, administration of potassium citrate (75 mg/kg administered with food twice daily) increased urine pH but had no effect on urinary calcium oxalate RSS in most dogs [76]. In the same study, administration of potassium citrate significantly reduced urinary calcium oxalate RSS in three Miniature Schnauzers, a breed known to be predisposed to calcium oxalate uroliths. In a grade I study of human patients with calcium oxalate nephroliths, administration of potassium-magnesium citrate daily for 3 years decreased urolith recurrence by 85% compared with placebo [77]. Effects of potassium citrate alone on urinary calcium oxalate saturation or urolith recurrence have not been evaluated in healthy cats or cats with calcium oxalate uroliths. Potassium citrate is found in one therapeutic food (Hill's Prescription Diet x/d Feline) that has been evaluated in cats with calcium oxalate uroliths [71].

Recommendations
- Consider using potassium citrate in cats that have recurrent calcium oxalate uroliths despite being fed a therapeutic food. Doses of 50 to 75 mg/kg administered by mouth every 12 hours with food have been recommended.
- Monitor urinalyses to detect calcium oxalate crystals, and adjust treatment to prevent their occurrence.

Evidence
The best evidence supporting these recommendations comes from human studies, epidemiologic studies in cats, one study in cats with calcium oxalate uroliths, and pathophysiologic rationale (grades II/III [Hill's Prescription Diet x/d Feline, which contains potassium citrate] and III/IV [potassium citrate alone]).

Thiazide Diuretics

Thiazide diuretics are known to cause renal tubular reabsorption of calcium, resulting in decreased urine calcium excretion, which may decrease the likelihood of urolith recurrence. Treatment with thiazides has been associated with significant reductions in recurrence of calcium oxalate uroliths in human patients [78,79]. In a study of normal dogs, chlorothiazide did not decrease urinary calcium excretion; however, hydrochlorothiazide significantly decreased urine calcium concentration and excretion in dogs with a history of calcium oxalate uroliths [80,81]. In a blind, crossover, controlled study of healthy cats, administration of hydrochlorothiazide suspension (1 mg/kg administered by mouth every 12 hours) was associated with significantly decreased urinary saturation of calcium oxalate compared with placebo. Potential side effects of thiazide diuretics include hypercalcemia and dehydration.

Recommendations
- For cats with recurrent calcium oxalate uroliths despite feeding moist therapeutic food and using potassium citrate, consider using thiazide diuretics (1–2 mg/kg administered by mouth every 12 hours).
- Carefully monitor cats receiving thiazides for dehydration and inappetence.
- Do not use thiazide diuretics in cats with hypercalcemia.

Evidence
The best evidence supporting these recommendations comes from pathophysiologic rationale, human studies, and one study in healthy cats (grade III/IV).

Vitamin B$_6$
Oxidation of glyoxylate results in formation of oxalate; however, a portion of glyoxylate is transaminated to glycine, a process that requires vitamin B$_6$ (pyridoxine) as a cofactor. It is possible that increased amounts of vitamin B$_6$ could drive the transamination reaction toward glycine, resulting in decreased amounts of oxalate, which may decrease the likelihood of calcium oxalate urolith formation [59]. In a large epidemiologic study of women, vitamin B$_6$ intake (>40 mg/d) was associated with a lower risk of urolith formation [82]. Increases in urinary oxalic acid excretion have been observed in kittens fed pyridoxine-deficient foods [83,84]. There have been no studies evaluating the effects of vitamin B$_6$ in cats with calcium oxalate uroliths, and because most commercially available pet foods are well supplemented with vitamin B$_6$, it seems unlikely that additional supplementation would be helpful. If a cat with calcium oxalate uroliths is being fed a homemade food, it would be appropriate to recommend supplementation with vitamin B$_6$.

Recommendations
- Most commercial cat foods contain adequate amounts of vitamin B$_6$, and additional supplementation is not needed.
- If a cat with calcium oxalate uroliths is being fed a homemade food, supplement with vitamin B$_6$ (2–4 mg/kg administered by mouth once daily).

Evidence
The best evidence supporting these recommendations comes from pathophysiologic rationale and an epidemiologic study in women (grade IV).

Vitamin C
In addition to dietary intake, urinary oxalate is derived from endogenous metabolism of ascorbic acid (vitamin C) and amino acids, such as glycine and

Box 1: Summary of evidence for treatments used to manage cats with FLUTD

Feline idiopathic cystitis

Grade III

- Environmental enrichment/stress reduction
- Feeding moist food (eg, Royal Canin Veterinary Diet feline Urinary SO, other moist foods)
- Long-term treatment with amitriptyline for severe cases

Grade III/IV

- Feline facial pheromone

Grade IV

- Increased salt intake to stimulate urine dilution
- Additional methods to stimulate water intake
- Analgesics and nonsteroidal anti-inflammatory drugs during acute episodes
- GAGs (eg, pentosan polysulfate, glucosamine/chondroitin sulfate)
- Propantheline during acute episodes

Dissolution of struvite uroliths

Grade III

- Calculolytic foods (ie, Hill's Prescription Diet s/d Feline, Medi-Cal/Royal Canin Dissolution Formula)

Grade IV

- Other therapeutic foods formulated to dissolve uroliths

Prevention of struvite urolith or urethral plug recurrence

Grade III

- Hill's Prescription Diet s/d (for urethral plug prevention)

Grade IV

- Therapeutic foods formulated to prevent struvite disease

Decreasing risk for calcium oxalate uroliths

Grade II/III

- Hill's Prescription Diet x/d Feline

Grade III/IV

- Purina UR Urinary St/Ox Feline Formula
- Royal Canin Veterinary Diet feline Urinary SO
- Feeding moist foods
- Potassium citrate
- Thiazide diuretics

Grade IV

- Other therapeutic foods formulated to prevent calcium oxalate
- Feeding multiple meals
- Using other methods to increase water intake
- Vitamin B_6

glyoxylate [85]. For this reason, it has been recommended that excessive vitamin C be avoided in cats with calcium oxalate uroliths. In a controlled study of healthy cats fed differing amounts of vitamin C (40–193 mg/kg of food) for 4 weeks, there was no significant change in urinary oxalate excretion [86]. Effects of vitamin C supplementation have not been studied in cats with calcium oxalate uroliths.

Recommendations
- It is reasonable to avoid excessive vitamin C supplementation in cats with calcium oxalate uroliths.

Evidence
The best evidence supporting these recommendations comes from pathophysiologic rationale and a controlled clinical study in healthy cats (grade IV).

SUMMARY
Many treatments have been recommended for managing cats with FLUTD. Veterinarians making therapeutic decisions should consider the quality of evidence supporting a recommendation to use (or not use) a particular treatment for cats with FLUTD (Box 1). Whenever possible, recommendations should be based on results of randomized and well-controlled scientific studies performed in clinical patients with the spontaneously occurring disease of interest. In the absence of such studies, one is left to make the best recommendation possible with consideration of all information, including the quality of the evidence. At this time, additional studies are needed to evaluate evidence for many currently recommended treatments for cats with FLUTD.

References
[1] Bartges J. Lower urinary tract disease in geriatric cats. Proceedings of the 15th American College of Veterinary Internal Medicine Forum 1997;322–4.
[2] Kirk CA, Lund E, Armstrong P. Prevalence of lower urinary tract disorders of dogs and cats in the United States. Proceedings of Waltham International Symposium 2001;61.
[3] Lekcharoensuk C, Osborne CA, Lulich JP. Epidemiologic study of risk factors for lower urinary tract diseases in cats. J Am Vet Med Assoc 2001;218:1429–35.
[4] Gerber B, Boretti FS, Kley S, et al. Evaluation of clinical signs and causes of lower urinary tract disease in European cats. J Small Anim Pract 2005;46:571–7.
[5] Kruger JM, Osborne CA, Goyal SM, et al. Clinical evaluation of cats with lower urinary tract disease. J Am Vet Med Assoc 1991;199:211–6.
[6] Buffington CA, Chew DJ, Kendall MS, et al. Clinical evaluation of cats with nonobstructive urinary tract diseases. J Am Vet Med Assoc 1997;210:46–50.
[7] Lund H, Krontveit R, Sorum H, et al. Bacteriuria in feline lower urinary tract disorders (FLUTD). J Vet Intern Med 2005;19:935–6.
[8] McMahon LA, Elliott JE, Syme HM. Prevalence and risk factors for urinary tract infections in cats with chronic renal failure. British Small Animal Veterinary Association Congress Scientific Proceedings 2006;534.
[9] Lulich JD, Osborne CA, O'Brien RD, et al. Feline renal failure: questions, answers, questions. Compendium on Continuing Education for the Practicing Veterinarian 1992;14:127–53.

[10] Osborne CA, Caywood DD, Johnston GR, et al. Feline perineal urethrostomy: a potential cause of feline lower urinary tract disease. Vet Clin North Am Small Anim Pract 1996;26:535–49.

[11] Osborne CA, Caywood DD, Johnston GR, et al. Perineal urethrostomy versus dietary management in prevention of recurrent lower urinary tract disease. J Small Anim Pract 1991;32: 296–305.

[12] Osborne C, Lulich J. Changing trends in composition of feline uroliths and urethral plugs. Available at: www.dvmnews.com. 2006.

[13] Cannon AB, Westropp JL, Kass PH, et al. Trends in feline urolithiasis: 1985-2004. J Vet Intern Med 2006;20:785–6.

[14] Houston DM, Moore AE, Favrin MG, et al. Feline urethral plugs and bladder uroliths: a review of 5484 submissions 1998–2003. Can Vet J 2003;44:974–7.

[15] Polzin D, Lund E, Walter P. From journal to patient: evidence-based medicine. In: Bonagura JD, editor. Kirk's current veterinary therapy, small animal practice, vol. 13. Philadelphia: WB Saunders; 2000. p. 2–8.

[16] Roudebush P, Allen TA, Dodd CE, et al. Application of evidence-based medicine to veterinary clinical nutrition. J Am Vet Med Assoc 2004;224:1765–71.

[17] Rosenthal RC. Evidence-based medicine concepts. Vet Clin North Am Small Anim Pract 2004;34:1–6.

[18] Keene BW. Towards evidence-based veterinary medicine. J Vet Intern Med 2000;14: 118–9.

[19] Westropp JL, Buffington CAT, Chew D. Feline lower urinary tract disorders. In: Ettinger SJ, Feldman EC, editors. Textbook of veterinary internal medicine. Philadelphia: Elsevier; 2005. p. 1828–50.

[20] Kruger JM, Osborne CA. Outcomes of treatment of feline idiopathic cystitis: what is the evidence? Urolithiasis 2000;2000:CD-ROM.

[21] Westropp JL, Tony Buffington CA. Feline idiopathic cystitis: current understanding of pathophysiology and management. Vet Clin North Am Small Anim Pract 2004;34: 1043–55.

[22] Westropp JL, Buffington C, Chew D. Feline lower urinary tract diseases. In: Ettinger SJ, Feldman EC, editors. Textbook of veterinary internal medicine. 6th edition. Philadelphia: Elsevier Saunders; 2005. p. 1828–50.

[23] Laule G. Positive reinforcement training and environmental enrichment: enhancing animal well-being. J Am Vet Med Assoc 2003;223:969–73.

[24] The indoor cat initiative. Available at: www.vet.ohio-state.edu/indoorcat. 2007.

[25] Neilson JC. Feline house soiling: elimination and marking behaviors. Vet Clin North Am Small Anim Pract 2003;33:287–301.

[26] Buffington CA, Westropp JL, Chew DJ, et al. Clinical evaluation of multimodal environmental modification (MEMO) in the management of cats with idiopathic cystitis. J Feline Med Surg 2006;8:261–8.

[27] Burger IH, Smith PM. Effects of diet on the urine characteristics of the cat. Nutrition, malnutrition and dietetics in the dog and cat. Proceedings of an International Symposium 1987;71–3.

[28] Gaskell CJ. The role of fluid in the feline urological syndrome. In: Burger IH, Rivers JPW, editors. Nutrition of the dog and cat. Cambridge (UK): Cambridge University Press; 1989. p. 353–6.

[29] Kirschvink N, Lhoest E, Leemans J, et al. Effects of feeding frequency on water intake in cats. J Vet Intern Med 2005;19:476.

[30] Markwell PJ, Buffington CA, Chew DJ, et al. Clinical evaluation of commercially available urinary acidification diets in the management of idiopathic cystitis in cats. J Am Vet Med Assoc 1999;214:361–5.

[31] Osborne CA, Stevens JB. Urinalysis: a clinical guide to compassionate patient care. Yardley (PA): Veterinary Learning Systems; 1999. p. 77.

[32] Hawthorne AJ, Markwell PJ. Dietary sodium promotes increased water intake and urine volume in cats. J Nutr 2004;134:2128S–9S.

[33] Devois C, Biourge V, Morice G. Influence of various amounts of dietary NaCl on urinary Na, Ca, and oxalate concentrations and excretions in adult cats. Proceedings of 10th European Society of Veterinary Internal Medicine Congress 2000;85.

[34] Luckschander N, Iben C, Hosgood G, et al. Dietary NaCl does not affect blood pressure in healthy cats. J Vet Intern Med 2004;18:463–7.

[35] Kirk CA, Jewell DE, Lowry SR. Effects of sodium chloride on selected parameters in cats. Veterinary Therapeutics 2006;7:333–46.

[36] Biourge VC, Devois C, Morice G, et al. Increased dietary NaCl significantly increases urine volume but does not increase urinary calcium oxalate and relative supersaturation in healthy cats. J Vet Intern Med 2001;15:301.

[37] Biourge VC. Sodium, urine dilution and lower urinary tract disease. 24th Annual American College of Veterinary Internal Medicine Forum 2006;17–9.

[38] Brown SA. Sodium and renal disease. 24th Annual American College of Veterinary Internal Medicine Forum 2006;13–4.

[39] National Research Council. Nutrient requirements of dogs and cats. Washington, DC: The National Academies Press; 2006.

[40] Buranakarl C, Mathur S, Brown SA. Effects of dietary sodium chloride intake on renal function and blood pressure in cats with normal and reduced renal function. Am J Vet Res 2004;65:620–7.

[41] Hughes KL, Slater MR, Geller S, et al. Diet and lifestyle variables as risk factors for chronic renal failure in pet cats. Prev Vet Med 2002;55:1–15.

[42] Ross SJ, Osborne CA, Kirk CA, et al. Clinical evaluation of effects of dietary modification for treatment of spontaneous chronic kidney disease in cats. J Am Vet Med Assoc 2006;229: 949–57.

[43] Chew DJ, Buffington CA, Kendall MS, et al. Amitriptyline treatment for severe recurrent idiopathic cystitis in cats. J Am Vet Med Assoc 1998;213:1282–6.

[44] Kruger JM, Conway TS, Kaneene JB, et al. Randomized controlled trial of the efficacy of short-term amitriptyline administration for treatment of acute, nonobstructive, idiopathic lower urinary tract disease in cats. J Am Vet Med Assoc 2003;222:749–58.

[45] Kraijer M, Fink-Gremmels J, Nickel RF. The short-term clinical efficacy of amitriptyline in the management of idiopathic feline lower urinary tract disease: a controlled clinical study. J Feline Med Surg 2003;5:191–6.

[46] Lukban JC, Whitmore KE, Sant GR. Current management of interstitial cystitis. Urol Clin North Am 2002;29:649–60.

[47] Osborne CA, Kruger JM, Lulich JP, et al. Prednisolone therapy of idiopathic feline lower urinary tract disease: a double-blind clinical study. Vet Clin North Am Small Anim Pract 1996;26:563–9.

[48] Griffith C, Steigerwalk E, Buffington C. Effects of a synthetic facial pheromone on behavior of cats. J Am Vet Med Assoc 2002;217:1154–6.

[49] Gunn-Moore DA, Cameron ME. A pilot study using synthetic feline facial pheromone for the management of feline idiopathic cystitis. J Feline Med Surg 2004;6:133–8.

[50] Palylyk-Colwell E. Chondroitin sulfate for interstitial cystitis. Issues in Emerging Health Technologies 2006;1–4.

[51] Anderson VR, Perry CM. Pentosan polysulfate: a review of its use in the relief of bladder pain or discomfort in interstitial cystitis. Drugs 2006;66:821–35.

[52] Gunn-Moore DA, Shenoy CM. Oral glucosamine and the management of feline idiopathic cystitis. J Feline Med Surg 2004;6:219–25.

[53] Barsanti JA, Finco DR, Shotts EB, et al. Feline urologic syndrome: further investigation into therapy. J Am Anim Hosp Assoc 1982;18:387–90.

[54] Osborne CA, Lulich JP, Kruger JM, et al. Medical dissolution of feline struvite urocystoliths. J Am Vet Med Assoc 1990;196:1053–63.

[55] Houston DM, Rinkardt NE, Hilton J. Evaluation of the efficacy of a commercial diet in the dissolution of feline struvite bladder uroliths. Vet Ther 2004;5:187–201.

[56] Abood SK, Zhang P, Ballam JM, et al. Relative supersaturation of struvite and calcium oxalate in urine from healthy cats. J Vet Intern Med 2000;14:353.

[57] Smith BH, Stevenson AE, Markwell PJ. Urinary relative supersaturations of calcium oxalate and struvite in cats are influenced by diet. J Nutr 1998;128:2763S–4S.

[58] Robertson WG, Jones JS, Heaton MA, et al. Predicting the crystallization potential of urine from cats and dogs with respect to calcium oxalate and magnesium ammonium phosphate (struvite). J Nutr 2002;132:1637S–41S.

[59] Allen TA, Kruger JM, et al. Feline lower urinary tract disease. In: Hand MS, Thatcher CD, Remillard RL, editors. Small animal clinical nutrition. Topeka (KS): Mark Morris Institute; 2000. p. 689–723.

[60] Devois C, Biourge V, Morice G, et al. Struvite and oxalate activity product ratios and crystalluria in cats fed acidifying diets. Urolithiasis 2000;2000:821–2.

[61] Xu H, Laflamme DP, Bartges JW, et al. Effect of dietary sodium on urine characteristics in healthy adult cats. J Vet Intern Med 2006;20:738.

[62] Bartges JW, Tarver SL, Schneider C. Comparison of struvite activity product ratios and relative supersaturations in urine collected from healthy cats consuming four struvite management diets. Proceedings Purina Nutrition Forum 1998;58–9.

[63] Stevenson AE, Wrigglesworth DJ, Markwell PJ. Urine pH and urinary relative supersaturation in healthy adult cats. Urolithiasis 2000;2000:818–20.

[64] Bovee K, Reif J, Maguire T, et al. Recurrence of feline urethral obstruction. J Am Vet Med Assoc 1979;174:93–6.

[65] Royal Canin product guide, 2006.

[66] Bartges JW, Kirk C, Lane IF. Update: management of calcium oxalate uroliths in dogs and cats. Vet Clin North Am Small Anim Pract 2004;34:969–87.

[67] Midkiff AM, Chew DJ, Randolph JF, et al. Idiopathic hypercalcemia in cats. J Vet Intern Med 2000;14:619–26.

[68] Savary KC, Price GS, Vaden SL. Hypercalcemia in cats: a retrospective study of 71 cases (1991–1997). J Vet Intern Med 2000;14:184–9.

[69] McClain HM, Barsanti JA, Bartges JW. Hypercalcemia and calcium oxalate urolithiasis in cats: a report of five cases. J Am Anim Hosp Assoc 1999;35:297–301.

[70] Kirk CA, Ling GV, Franti CE, et al. Evaluation of factors associated with development of calcium oxalate urolithiasis in cats. J Am Vet Med Assoc 1995;207:1429–34.

[71] Lulich JP, Osborne CA, Lekcharoensuk C, et al. Effects of diet on urine composition of cats with calcium oxalate urolithiasis. J Am Anim Hosp Assoc 2004;40:185–91.

[72] Robertson WG, Markwell PJ. Predicting the calcium oxalate crystallisation potential of cat urine. Waltham Focus 1999;9:32–3.

[73] Stevenson AE, Blackburn JM, Markwell PJ, et al. Nutrient intake and urine composition in calcium oxalate stone-forming dogs: comparison with healthy dogs and impact of dietary modification. Vet Ther 2004;5:218–31.

[74] Ross S, Osborne C, Polzin D. Epidemiology of feline nephroliths and ureteroliths. Proceedings 23rd American College of Veterinary Internal Medicine Forum 2005;746–7

[75] Lekcharoensuk C, Osborne CA, Lulich JP, et al. Association between dietary factors and calcium oxalate and magnesium ammonium phosphate urolithiasis in cats. J Am Vet Med Assoc 2001;219:1228–37.

[76] Stevenson AE, Wrigglesworth DJ, Smith BH, et al. Effects of dietary potassium citrate supplementation on urine pH and urinary relative supersaturation of calcium oxalate and struvite in healthy dogs. Am J Vet Res 2000;61:430–5.

[77] Ettinger B, Pak CY, Citron JT, et al. Potassium-magnesium citrate is an effective prophylaxis against recurrent calcium oxalate nephrolithiasis. J Urol 1997;158:2069–73.

[78] Pearle MS, Roehrborn CG, Pak CY. Meta-analysis of randomized trials for medical prevention of calcium oxalate nephrolithiasis. J Endourol 1999;13:679–85.

[79] Fernandez-Rodriguez A, Arrabal-Martin M, Garcia-Ruiz MJ, et al. The role of thiazides in the prophylaxis of recurrent calcium lithiasis. Actas Urol Esp 2006;30:305–9 [in Spanish].

[80] Lulich JP, Osborne CA. Effects of chlorothiazide on urinary excretion of calcium in clinically normal dogs. Am J Vet Res 1992;53:2328–32.

[81] Lulich JP, Osborne CA, Lekcharoensuk C, et al. Effects of hydrochlorothiazide and diet in dogs with calcium oxalate urolithiasis. J Am Vet Med Assoc 2001;218:1583–6.

[82] Curhan GC, Willett WC, Speizer FE, et al. Intake of vitamins B6 and C and the risk of kidney stones in women. J Am Soc Nephrol 1999;10:840–5.

[83] Bai SC, Sampson DA, Morris JG, et al. The level of dietary protein affects the vitamin B-6 requirement of cats. J Nutr 1991;121:1054–61.

[84] Bai SC, Sampson DA, Morris JG, et al. Vitamin B-6 requirement of growing kittens. J Nutr 1989;119:1020–7.

[85] Osborne CA, Bartges JW, Lulich JP, et al. Canine urolithiasis. In: Hand MS, Thatcher CD, Remillard RL, et al, editors. Small animal clinical nutrition. Topeka (KS): Mark Morris Institute; 2000. p. 605–88.

[86] Yu S, Gross KL. Moderate dietary vitamin C supplement does not affect urinary oxalate concentration in cats. J Anim Physiol Anim Nutr 2005;89:428.

Vet Clin Small Anim 37 (2007) 559–577

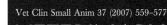

VETERINARY CLINICS
SMALL ANIMAL PRACTICE

Evidence-Based Wound Management: A Systematic Review of Therapeutic Agents to Enhance Granulation and Epithelialization

Maria A. Fahie, DVM, MS[a,b],*, Donna Shettko, DVM[c],*

[a]Small Animal Surgery, Western University of Health Sciences, College of Veterinary Medicine, 309 East Second Street, Pomona, CA 91766, USA
[b]Orange Veterinary Hospital, Orange, CA, USA
[c]Equine Surgery, Western University of Health Sciences, College of Veterinary Medicine, 309 East Second Street, Pomona, CA 91766, USA

Successful management of open wounds in dogs requires knowledge of the physiology of wound healing and application of that knowledge to choose appropriate therapeutic intervention. Open wound management is considered to include wounds healing by second intention, or contraction and epithelialization. Such wounds are commonly managed in veterinary practice and can occur as a result of degloving injuries, bite trauma, burns, surgical wound dehiscence, or resective oncologic surgery.

The human and veterinary literature describes the conceptual division of wound healing into three stages: inflammation, proliferation, and maturation. These stages are described in detail elsewhere [1,2], summarized in Fig. 1, and illustrated in Figs. 2–4. Inflammation is a vascular and cellular response to injury that initially involves vasoconstriction to control hemorrhage and then vasodilation to enhance the wound site with a transudative fluid. Transudate components influencing wound healing include leukocytes, plasma proteins, complement, antibodies, water, electrolytes, and humoral substances. Important components in the second-intention wound healing process include mast cells [3] and growth factors [4,5]. Subcutaneous tissue also plays a role because its removal from surgically created full-thickness wounds in dogs is reported to reduce wound perfusion, granulation, contraction, epithelialization, and overall healing [6]. Granulation tissue formation is the ultimate goal of the inflammatory stage to help it progress to the proliferative phase. For normal healing, the processes of cell production, cell death, capillary

*Corresponding authors. Western University of Health Sciences, College of Veterinary Medicine, 309 East Second Street, Pomona, CA 91766. *E-mail addresses:* mfahie@westernu.edu (M.A. Fahie); dshettko@westernu.edu (D. Shettko).

0195-5616/07/$ – see front matter
doi:10.1016/j.cvsm.2007.02.001

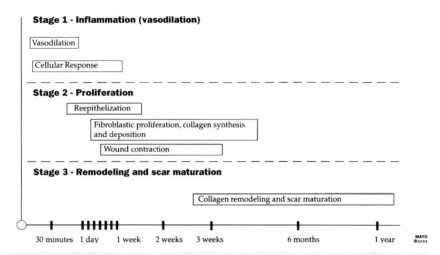

Fig. 1. Summary of the three stages of wound healing. (*From* Sherris DA, Kern EB. Essential surgical skills. 2nd edition. Philadelphia: WB Saunders; 2004. p. 15. By permission of Mayo Foundation for Medical Education and Research. All rights reserved.)

formation/obliteration, and collagen production/hydrolysis/degradation/ absorption must all be balanced in the proliferative phase. Epithelial migration and proliferation are initiated and progress by contact inhibition and contact guidance. During maturation, collagen is continuously remodeled to become

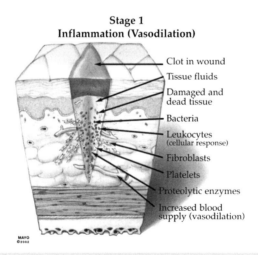

Fig. 2. Human epidermis and dermis with components of wound healing that are similar for dogs. Stage 1 inflammation (vasodilation). (*From* Sherris DA, Kern EB. Essential surgical skills. 2nd edition. Philadelphia: WB Saunders; 2004. p. 13. By permission of Mayo Foundation for Medical Education and Research. All rights reserved.)

Stage 2
Proliferation

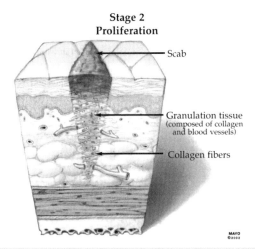

Fig. 3. Human epidermis and dermis with components of wound healing that are similar for dogs. Stage 2 proliferation. (*From* Sherris DA, Kern EB. Essential surgical skills. 2nd edition. Philadelphia: WB Saunders; 2004. p. 14. By permission of Mayo Foundation for Medical Education and Research. All rights reserved.)

structurally superior. Epithelial structures, such as hair follicles and sebaceous glands, can appear after complete wound re-epithelialization.

Stages of wound healing are intertwined processes, and it may be possible to have a therapeutic agent that enhances one stage although inhibiting another. For example, an occlusive dressing facilitates a moist wound environment and retention of wound fluid and its various components that may enhance healing.

Stage 3
Scar Maturation

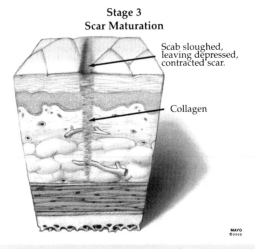

Fig. 4. Human epidermis and dermis with components of wound healing that are similar for dogs. Stage 3 scar maturation. (*From* Sherris DA, Kern EB. Essential surgical skills. 2nd edition. Philadelphia: WB Saunders; 2004. p. 15; with permission.)

Conversely, it keeps oxygen away from the tissues, and oxygen is important in collagen synthesis [7]. In some studies, a particular therapeutic agent enhances wound epithelialization but the percentage of wound contraction and total wound healing are not significantly different [8,9]. One of the authors, who has published much research in wound healing, makes the following general statement about his research: "If a factor has an effect on open wound healing, whether positive or negative, that effect is most marked early during the course of healing (first 10–15 days). After that, differences between treatment and control wounds are negligible."

The bacterial organisms anticipated to be present within a wound or to become present within a wound during open wound management include *Staphylococcus aureus*, β-hemolytic *Streptococcus*, *Staphylococcus epidermidis*, α-hemolytic *Streptococcus*, *Escherichia coli*, and *Proteus* sp [7,10]. Any antibiotics that decrease blood monocytes or tissue macrophages, interfere with fibroblast migration or differentiation, or interfere with protein synthesis activity could theoretically inhibit wound healing [11].

In the human medical field, results of a recent *Cochrane Database of Systematic Reviews* found that there was " insufficient evidence to suggest whether the choice of dressing or topical agent affects the healing of surgical wounds healing by secondary intention" [12]. After analysis of our literature review, the same statement seems to apply to wound healing in dogs. Many agents are commercially available for use in open wound management, but evidence in the form of quality reliable veterinary research may be lacking. At least once source recently stated that veterinary informatics is an embryonic field [13]. Another complicating factor is that based on previous studies, it is difficult to ensure that in vitro or alternate species study results can be applied accurately and reliably to dogs [14,15]. Some in vitro studies may not have the same result in vivo. For example, there is a level 1b grade A (Table 1) in vivo study comparing wound lavage with sterile water versus chlorhexidine that did not demonstrate a significant difference in wound healing [16]. In contrast, a level 4 grade C (see Table 1) in vitro study did show a difference [17]. Recently, significant

Table 1
Levels of evidence

Level	Grade	Study type
1a	A	SR with homogeneity of RCTs
1b	A	Individual RCT with narrow confidence interval
2a	B	SR with homogeneity of cohort studies
2b	B	Individual cohort study
3a	B	SR with homogeneity of case-control studies
4	C	Case series, in vitro studies
5	D	Expert opinion

Abbreviations: RCT, randomized controlled trial; SR, systematic review.
From Oxford Centre for Evidence-Based Medicine Levels of Evidence. 2001. Available at: www.cebm.net/levels_of_evidence.asp. Accessed April 16, 2006.

species differences in second-intention cutaneous wound healing processes have also been reported, with cats healing more slowly than dogs [18].

Interpretation and application of results of those quality studies that exist in the veterinary literature to current clinical cases can be impaired by several factors. The position of the wound on the dog's body has an effect on the process of wound healing. One study found that wounds more proximally located on the trunk healed more slowly [7]. There could be a difference between healing time for a patient's traumatically induced wound compared with a surgically created full-thickness open wound. Traumatic wounds could have significant impairment of local tissue vascular supply and increased contamination. The advancement of techniques to measure wound healing objectively may make it difficult to compare older studies with more recent research. Most earlier studies objectively measure wound healing by hand tracing or digital photography, followed by wound digitizing with computer software and calculation of parameters of interest [7,10]. Histopathologic examination is also used. Some more recent studies use laser Doppler perfusion imaging (LDPI) as a quantitative evaluation of tissue perfusion at the wound site [8,19]. Quantification of hydroxyproline content within a wound granulation bed is also described as an advancement to determine specific collagen type within healing wounds [20]. If those more objective measures were available in earlier studies, results and conclusions may have been different.

The authors' objective was to investigate whether or not there are any available therapeutic agents that enhance granulation or epithelialization of open wounds in dogs. The criteria for inclusion in this study were the following: canine patients, research or statements published in veterinary journals, and surgically created and traumatic full-thickness wounds healing by second intention.

METHODS
Search Strategy
An electronic bibliographic search was performed using the PubMed database and Veterinary Information Network [21] in April 2006. A broad query was done, and the following user string acts as an example for all agents: (canine) and (hydrogel) and (wound). Once several studies were identified, common authors were noted; a search by author name was also performed using, for example, "Swaim, S."

This systematic analysis was restricted to veterinary literature that included canine patients with surgically created or traumatic wounds healing by second intention. Literature that satisfied inclusion criteria was reviewed independently by the authors, who were assessing quality of study design, details of interventions, and outcome measures. Literature was assigned an appropriate level of evidence and grade for reference based on the Oxford Centre for Evidence-Based Medicine recommendations [22] (see Table 1). The hierarchy of evidence has also been displayed as a pyramid by the Medical Research Library of Brooklyn [23], with in vitro research at the base of the pyramid, followed consecutively by animal research, ideas/editorials/opinions, research in other species, case reports, case series, case-control studies, cohort studies, randomized controlled studies and, finally, systematic reviews at the top of the pyramid.

Results and conclusions are interpreted similarly to a model used in a systematic review of veterinary dermatologic literature [24], which modified the strength of recommendation qualifier from the 1996 report of the US Preventive Services Task Force [25]. Statements regarding the level of evidence (good, fair, or insufficient) and the agent or procedure tested (for or against its use) are made.

RESULTS

Most level 1b studies showed no significant difference in overall wound contraction and epithelialization. There may be differences between groups on certain days, but, overall, no difference is noted. Table 2 summarizes attributes of some level 1b studies used to assign the study level and grade.

Wound Lavage Solutions

Literature was identified for the following wound lavage solutions: povidone iodine, chlorhexidine diacetate, 3% hydrogen peroxide, 0.9% sodium chloride (NaCl), lactated Ringer's solution (LRS), normal saline, phosphate-buffered saline (PBS), tap water, and Dakin's solution (0.125%–0.5% sodium hypochlorite).

A level 1b grade A study was performed to compare previously reported in vitro effects of 0.0005% and 0.05% chlorhexidine diacetate and 0.1% and 1.0% povidone-iodine concentrations with effects on in vivo wound healing [14]. In the in vitro (level 4 grade C) study [26], 0.05% chlorhexidine diacetate and 1% povidone iodine were cytotoxic to canine fibroblasts. The in vivo study found that the 0.05% chlorhexidine diacetate had significantly more bactericidal activity compared with the povidone-iodine and saline control groups. Chlorhexidine also had a 6-hour residual activity level not found in the povidone-iodine group. Wound contraction and epithelialization were similar in the chlorhexidine- and povidone-iodine–treated wounds. These results suggested that concentrations of chlorhexidine diacetate that are cytotoxic to fibroblasts in vitro do not interfere with wound healing in vivo.

A level 1b grade A study compared the effects of four preparations of 0.05% chlorhexidine diacetate on wound healing in dogs [16]. Chlorhexidine was diluted to 0.05% in sterile water, in 0.9% NaCl, in LRS, and in LRS that was allowed to form precipitate. All 0.05% chlorhexidine solutions were 100% bactericidal. There was no difference between groups with regard to wound contraction and epithelialization. The LRS/chlorhexidine diacetate precipitate group did not have impaired wound healing or reduced antimicrobial effects [10].

A level 4 grade C in vitro study compared the effects of PBS (control group), sterile tap water, normal saline, and LRS on canine fibroblasts [17]. Effects were

Table 2
Summary of attributes used to assign study level and grade

Citation (reference)	Morgan and colleagues [7]	Ramsey and colleagues [10]	Swaim and colleagues [8]	Scardino and colleagues [9]
Quality of evidence	Level 1b grade A	Level 1b grade A	Level 1b grade A	Level 1b grade A
Randomization	Yes	Yes	Yes	Yes
Masking of outcome assessor	Unclear	Unclear	Unclear	Unclear
No. dogs entered in trial	10	12	9	12
No. wounds per dog	6	4	4	3
Length of trial	28 days	28 days	51 days	21 days
Topical agent	Occlusive (hydrogel and hydrocolloid), polyethylene semiocclusive	Equine amnion, hydrogel, polyethylene, Release	Occlusive hydrolyzed bovine collagen	Pulsed electromagnetic field
Outcome measures	Bacterial culture, digitized tracing, histopathologic examination; ANOVA and Duncan's multiple range test, $P<.05$	Photographs of wound digitized, ANOVA, (Kruskal-Wallis one-way)	Subjective wound evaluation, percentage of tissue perfusion by laser Doppler perfusion imaging, planimetry, histopathologic examination, paired t test, Wilcoxon paired sample test	Digitized tracing (planimetry), histopathologic examination, Shapiro-Wilk W statistic, P value, normal probability plot Wilcoxon ranked sum, Fisher's exact test, all $P<.05$

measured at 30, 60, and 150 seconds and at 5 and 10 minutes. Sterile tap water damaged cells at all times, probably because of alkaline pH, hypotonicity, and, possibly, cytotoxic trace elements. Normal saline caused problems after 10 minutes, probably because of the acidic pH. LRS caused no problems. This study suggests PBS and LRS do not induce fibroblast injury, whereas normal saline and tap water cause mild and severe cytotoxicity, respectively.

Level 5 grade D expert opinions of three surgeons state that hydrogen peroxide and sodium hypochlorite solutions are cytotoxic to fibroblasts, delay epithelialization, and are not recommended as wound lavage solutions [1,27–29].

Topical Antimicrobial Agents

Few studies were found in the veterinary literature regarding topical antimicrobial agents for open wound management, and the issue is controversial. Can prophylactic use of antimicrobials lead to infection with a resistant organism? In infected wounds, is oral or topical administration preferred? Certainly, the presence of wound infection would delay wound healing; however, topical antimicrobial agents can have deleterious effects on wound contraction, granulation, and epithelialization. The potential benefit of the antimicrobial effect could theoretically be outweighed by the risks associated with impaired wound healing.

Gentamicin sulfate (Garamycin; Schering Plough Corporation, Kenilworth, New Jersey) may be especially good for *Pseudomonas* infection, but certain formulations, including the cream base (0.1% gentamicin cream), can adversely affect wound contraction and epithelialization. A level 1b grade A study found that gentamicin solution (0.1%) was preferable compared with the cream, because the latter initially resulted in wound enlargement rather than contraction [11,28]. By 14 and 21 days, however, there was no significant difference in epithelialization. A relatively recent study uses topical 0.1% Garamycin ointment as a standard wound care protocol in all treatment groups [19].

Bacitracin zinc, neomycin sulfate, and polymyxin B sulfate (BNP; Neosporin, Burroughs Wellcome Company, Research Triangle Park, North Carolina; Vetrobiotic, Pharmaderm, Melville, New York) ointment has a broad spectrum of antimicrobial activity. BNP is reported to lack cytotoxic effects on fibroblasts in vitro and to have enhanced epithelialization of partial-thickness wounds in pigs by 25% [11]. The zinc component of this combination product is reported to have a potential positive effect on epithelialization but a potential negative effect on wound contraction [30]. In a level 1b grade A study of open pad wounds, BNP was compared with aloe vera extract gel containing allantoin and acemannan (Dermal wound gel; Allerderm, Fort Worth, Texas). At 7 days, BNP and control wounds had actually increased in size and the aloe vera gel group had a smaller unhealed wound area. At 14 and 21 days, there was no difference between groups [31]. Level 5 grade D expert opinions report positive results with topical application of BNP [27,28].

Silver sulfadiazine 1% (Silvadene; Marion Labs, Kansas City, Missouri) has broad antimicrobial activity against most gram-positive and gram-negative bacteria and most fungi. It is widely used for open wounds induced by burn trauma in human beings. It is reported to have enhanced re-epithelialization in pig wounds by 28% [28]. It is also reported to be toxic to human keratinocytes and fibroblasts in vitro [30]. No veterinary studies of its effect on wound healing were identified in our literature search.

A level 4 grade C report of 54 dogs treated with topical furazolium chloride had no objective measures of wound healing but concluded subjectively that 90% of dogs had excellent or good results [32]. Nitrofurazone (Furacin; Smith Kline Beecham Pharmaceuticals, Philadelphia, Pennsylvania) is reported in a level 5 grade D expert opinion paper to have slowed the re-epithelialization process in pig partial-thickness wounds by 30% [28].

WOUND DRESSINGS
Hydrocolloid Occlusive Dressings
Hydrocolloid dressings are occlusive type dressings that inhibit contamination, stimulate collagen synthesis, and reduce fluid loss from wounded tissues, promoting a moist wound healing environment [7]. The occlusive dressings resulted in more exuberant granulation tissue present and more positive bacterial cultures. A level 1b grade A study compared hydrocolloid and hydrogel occlusive dressings with polyethylene semiocclusive dressings [7]. In all three groups, there was no significant difference in wound healing at days 4 and 7. The exudate underneath the hydrocolloid dressing was malodorous, tenacious, and difficult to remove during the bandage changes. In the wounds treated with hydrocolloid dressings, no statistically significant differences were measured in mean percentage of contraction or new epithelialization on day 21 or day 28 after surgery [7]. They also had significantly less total wound area healed on days 21 (5 of 13 wounds) and 28 (7 of 14 wounds) after surgery and significantly fewer wounds more than 90% healed on day 28 [7].

In a level 4 grade C study of 15 dogs with burns, all managed with hydrocolloid dressings (Granuflex; ConvaTec Limited Harrington House, Uxbridge, The Netherlands), the wounds healed well and did not require grafting [33]. A level 5 grade D expert opinion suggests that hydrocolloid dressings are occlusive and may prolong wound contraction [34].

Polyethylene Semiocclusive Dressings
The literature search identified two studies investigating semiocclusive rayon/polyethylene (Telfa Adhesive Pads; Kendall Healthcare Products Company, Mansfield, Massachusetts) and polyethylene (Melolite; Smith & Nephew, Largo, Florida). One study looked at full-thickness skin wounds on the forelimbs of dogs [7], whereas the other study examined wounds located on the dorsum of dogs [10].

When looking at the polyethylene on postoperative days 14, 21, and 28, the wounds had significantly more new epithelium covering them [7]. By postoperative day 21, 13 of 14 wounds under the polyethylene were healed, and by day 28 after surgery, 100% were healed [7]. The polyethylene semiocclusive dressing group had a significantly higher mean percentage of re-epithelialization compared with both occlusive dressings (described in the previous section on hydrocolloid dressings) at days 14, 21, and 28 [7].

The other study compared transparent polyethylene sheeting and a semiocclusive rayon/polyethylene [10]. The polyethylene sheeting developed a moderate to extreme amount of purulent exudate after day 3. Seventeen wounds were completely healed in 23 or fewer days, although none of the wounds had healed in the polyethylene group. By day 28, only 41% of the wounds treated with semiocclusive rayon/polyethylene and 16% of those treated with polyethylene sheeting had healed. The conclusion drawn is that the transparent polyethylene sheeting cannot be recommended for the initial treatment of full-thickness wounds [10].

Hydrogel

Hydrogel occlusive dressings are available as gel pastes or as composite sheets consisting of the hydrogel adhered to a thin fine-mesh synthetic sheet. Hydrogel is composed of insoluble hydrophilic polymers. Hydrogel dressings (BioDres, DVM Pharmaceuticals, Miami, Florida; Curity Conforma Gel, Kendall Canada, Peterborough, Ontario, Canada) enhanced granulation tissue and wound contraction [7] compared with hydrocolloid and polyethylene in the level 1b grade A study described in the preceding hydrocolloid section. At postoperative days 21 and 28, the forelimb wounds under the hydrogel dressing were significantly different, with a greater mean percentage of wound contraction. The wounds covered with hydrogel had a greater percentage of wound healing by contraction, as exhibited by the ratio of contraction to epithelialization, which was significantly larger for wounds treated with the hydrogel on postoperative days 21 and 28. Because contraction is related to the production and maturation of granulation tissue, the hydrogel dressing favored granulation tissue and rapid wound contraction. By postoperative day 28, the mean percentage of wound healing was 98.04% ± 0.78% [7]. The study concludes that hydrogel dressings are preferred, because healing was primarily by wound contraction, resulting in a smaller scar [7].

The other study (level 1b grade A) does not recommend the use of hydrogel for the initial treatment of full-thickness wounds but states that occlusive dressings may be more beneficial for the treatment of full-thickness wounds in the reparative stage [10]. This study noted that slight to moderate amounts of purulent serosanguineous or purulent exudate might occur on the wound surface. The percentage of wounds completely healed by day 25 was 25% and remained at 25% by the end of the study (day 28) [10].

An expert opinion (level 5 grade D) suggests the use of this dressing to enhance wound contraction, angiogenesis, and wound epithelialization [33–35]. The Veterinary Information Network [21] has a thread describing successful wound healing with BioDres. A cost estimate for this product is $4 to $5 for one 7-cm × 10-cm sheet.

Polyurethane Foam

Polyurethane foam dressings (Allevyn; Smith & Nephew) are nonadherent and quite absorbent. Expert opinion (level 5 grade D) states that these are extremely absorbent and nonadherent and that they stimulate granulation tissue [35].

Nonadherent Dressings

Only one study (level 1b, grade A) compared four nonadherent dressings of rayon/polyethylene (Telfa Adhesive Pads; Kendall Healthcare Products Company), cotton nonadherent film dressing, fine-mesh gauze petrolatum, and commercial petrolatum emulsion [36]. The dressings were applied to small full-thickness skin defects on the dorsum of 12 dogs. Regardless of the dressing used, all the wounds contracted rapidly from day 0 to day 14, followed by slower contraction from day 14 to day 21. By day 14, there was no significant difference between all four dressings. At day 21, wounds treated with rayon/polyethylene and cotton nonadherent film dressings had a significantly greater mean percentage of epithelialization than did the wounds treated with petrolatum.

The cotton had a significantly less mean percentage of wound contraction by day 7 than petrolatum [36]. Wound epithelialization developed rapidly from 1 to 3 weeks. At day 7, the mean percentage of epithelialization for the wounds treated with the cotton nonadherent film dressing was significantly greater than that for wounds treated with the petrolatum products. Yet, by day 14, a statistically significant difference was not identified [36].

The two petrolatum products, fine-mesh gauze petrolatum dressings and commercial petrolatum emulsion dressings, caused some minor hemorrhage during dressing removal during the first week of treatment [36]. These two dressings allowed more absorption of exudate than cotton. The commercial petrolatum emulsion dressings had a significantly higher mean percentage of contraction by day 7 than the rayon/polyethylene and cotton dressings. In addition, the mean percentage of contraction was significantly higher than in the wounds treated with rayon/polyethylene dressings, but a statistical significance did not exist after day 7. Epithelialization of wounds treated with the petrolatum dressings or the commercial petrolatum dressings developed slowly during the first week [36].

Lee and colleagues [36] summarize their results with the following statements, because the four nonadherent dressing materials had different properties that affected different factors of wound healing. When a wound has newly formed granulation tissue and exudate is present, a nonadherent contact dressing with open mesh should be used. Yet, when a wound has healthy granulation tissue and serosanguineous drainage and is starting to epithelialize, a nonadherent petrolatum-free dressing should be used [36].

Equine Amnion Dressing

Equine amnion is an occlusive dressing that prevents fluid, protein, and electrolyte losses from the wound; decreases wound site pain; and promotes an earlier return to mobility [10]. It favored wound contraction and epithelialization compared with hydrogel and polyethylene nonadherent dressing in a level 1b grade

A study [10]. The study had 12 dogs with 2 full-thickness wounds created. Wounds were treated for 28 days and photographed on days 1, 3, 7, 14, 21, and 28. Bandages were changed daily for the first 5 days and subsequently on 2, 4, and 6 days of each week. The quantity of exudate was subjectively evaluated at each bandage change. Wound outlines, percentages of wound contraction and epithelialization, and total healing were calculated. Equine amnion provided good occlusion of the wounds, so the wounds remained moist under the contact layer of the dressing and bandages did not adhere to the wounds. Slight to moderate amounts of serosanguineous and purulent exudate were present under the bandage beginning on day 16. On days 14, 21, and 28, the mean percentage of wound healed and mean percentage of wound contraction were greater. Time to complete healing was significantly different between groups. Seventeen wounds were completely healed in 23 days. Eleven of the 17 wounds were in the amnion group. The mean time to complete (100%) healing for the wounds bandaged with amnion was 21 days. Ramsey and colleagues [10] concluded that amnion membrane dressing was superior to the other occlusive dressings in its ability to promote rapid wound healing.

Porcine Small Intestinal Submucosa Dressing

Porcine small intestinal submucosa (PSIS) is composed of collagen, fibronectin, hyaluronic acid, chondroitin sulfate A, heparin, heparin sulfate, and growth factors. A level 1b grade A study of dogs with open wounds and exposed metatarsal bone evaluated the effect of PSIS (Vetbiosist; Smiths Medical PM, Waukesha, Wisconsin) on healing time, epithelialization, angiogenesis, contraction, and inflammation [19]. Wound healing was monitored objectively using histopathologic examination, planimetry, and LDPI. There was not a significant difference noted in mean wound size between the control and treated wounds at day 7, with total wound healing almost completely attributable to wound contraction. On day 21, there was not a significant difference in the percentage of total wound healing, contraction, or epithelialization between the treated and control groups. At day 7, LDPI showed a significantly higher mean perfusion for the control wounds compared with treated wounds, yet there was not a significant difference between wound groups on days 14 and 21. Overall, the study showed no differences in healing between control wounds and wounds treated with PSIS [19].

A level 4 grade C case report describes successful healing of a canine open wound on the extremity when PSIS was applied [37]. A level 5 grade D report states that PSIS in a sheet form is a collagen dressing used to enhance healing by acting as a lattice for cell ingrowth [38]. Another level 5 grade D expert opinion reports that PSIS is a topical wound dressing that may act as a wound contraction inhibitor [34].

Hydrolyzed Bovine Collagen Dressings

Collagen is a key component in the proliferation/repair stage of wound healing [8]. Collagen applied to the wound can act as a template for fibroblasts to enter, resulting in newly synthesized endogenous collagen. The effects of hydrolyzed bovine collagen dressings were compared with those of semiocclusive nonadherent dressings [8]. The collagen dressing (FasCURE; Loveland Industry, Greeley, Colorado) was hydrophilic and enhanced a moist wound environment. When assessing LDPI, there was not a significant difference in epithelialization between treated and control wounds [8]. The mean percentages of wound contraction and total wound healing did not significantly differ between treated and control wounds at any time. Only on day 7 was the mean percentage of epithelialization significantly greater in the treated wounds [8]. There was no difference detected by histologic variables between the treated and control wounds. Swaim and colleagues [8] concluded that, clinically, the hydrolyzed bovine collagen dressing might be useful for the treatment of wounds in need of early epithelialization. Expert opinions (level 5 grade D) recommend the use of collagen dressings [33].

Calcium Alginate Dressings

This type of dressing interchanges its calcium content for sodium in the wound fluid to form a sodium alginate gel over the wound surface. It has hydrophilic properties, enhances granulation tissue formation, and may provide hemostasis. One available product is Dermacea Alginate (Sherwood Medical, St. Louis, Missouri). Expert opinion (level 5 grade D) states that this type of dressing should be used only on heavily to moderately exudative wounds [33].

OTHER THERAPEUTIC AGENTS/PROCEDURES

Chitosan

A level 1b grade A study of three dogs, each with eight wounds, evaluated chitosan (KITE-oh-zan) as an accelerator of wound healing [39]. Chitosan is a linear copolymer of linked β (1→4) glucosamine and N-acetyl-D-glucosamine derived from the chitin-rich crab shell. Chitosan is reported to enhance the functions of inflammatory cells, such as polymorphonuclear leukocytes (PMNs; phagocytosis and production of osteopontin and leukotriene B4), macrophages (phagocytosis and production of interleukin [IL]-1), transforming growth factor-β1 (TGF-β1), platelet-derived growth factor (PDGF), and fibroblasts (production of IL-8) [40]. A cotton fiber type of chitosan product was fabricated and used in the study. A commercially available chitosan dressing exists in the United States (HemCon; HemCon Medical Technologies, Inc., Portland, OR). Study results confirmed increased inflammatory cell infiltrate in the initial wound healing stage by histopathologic examination. Granulation tissue was more pronounced in treated wounds at days 9 and 15, and an excess of granulation tissue could impair epithelialization. Type III collagen production was increased based on the results of immunohistochemical typing.

An earlier level 1b grade A study comparing chitin, chitosan, and a control group found that, subjectively, re-epithelialization seemed greater in both treatment groups versus controls; however, when objectively statistically analyzed, there was no significant difference between the three groups [41].

Pulsed Electromagnetic Field

A pulsed electromagnetic field (PEMF) generates complex multiform pulses of oscillating electromagnetic fields in the ultralow frequency range (0.5–18 Hz) [9]. Magnetic field and low-intensity laser beam treatments can inhibit microbial flora and enhance wound healing. A level 1b grade A study evaluated the effects of PEMF on open wound healing. Objective wound healing assessment was performed using tensiometry, planimetry, LDPI, and histologic examination. At days 10 and 15, there was a significantly greater percentage of epithelialization; however, the percentage of reduction in wound size, percentage of total healing, and histologic scores were not significantly different at the end of the study [9]. One surgeon's level 5 grade D expert opinion suggests that this treatment modality be applied in cases requiring enhanced wound contraction [34].

Low-Intensity Laser Light

Photoirradiation is thought to stimulate healing by inducing cellular proliferation, collagen synthesis, growth factor release, and DNA synthesis [42]. A level 4 grade C case report of successful healing of a chronic extremity wound was found. The case report mentions two previously published case reports that, in contrast, did not note differences in healing.

Epidermal Growth Factor

Epidermal growth factor (EGF) is an amino-acid polypeptide that facilitates epidermal cell regeneration and stimulates proliferation and migration of keratinocytes [43]. In a level 1b grade A study, a gelatin film dressing with EGF was evaluated. Results revealed that the treatment group had greater re-epithelialization in four wounds on two dogs [43].

Three dogs with chronic perianal region wounds for more than 6 months were managed with an EGF-soaked dressing, and the wounds in two of the dogs healed within 24 and 35 days [44].

Sugar

Sugar has antibacterial action and accelerates wound healing by enhanced tissue formation and epithelialization [45]. Sugar dressings draw macrophages into the wound and accelerate sloughing of necrotic tissue. Sugar provides a local nutrient source, decreases inflammatory edema, and enhances sterilization of the wound, resulting in enhanced granulation and epithelialization [45]. Three case reports of traumatic wounds describe successful wound management with sugar dressings. The Veterinary Information Network [21] has several threads in which successful case management with sugar is described in cats and dogs.

Honey

Honey is reported to have a bactericidal effect by liberation of hydrogen peroxide. It also has a phytochemical constituent that enhances sterilization. It decreases inflammatory edema, attracts macrophages, accelerates necrotic tissue sloughing, provides a local cellular energy source, and forms a protective protein layer over the wound [46]. One successful level 4 grade C case report is described, but application of the honey required anesthesia because of vocalization/pain [46]. That complication was not found in any form of report. The Veterinary Information Network [21] has several threads, presumed to be level 5 expert opinions, wherein successful case management with honey is described in cats and dogs. It is suggested that sugar is better for wounds that have a defect into which it can be poured, whereas honey is better for flatter wound surfaces [46].

Hydrophilic Preparations

There were no level 3 studies identified for the following products; however, level 5 grade D expert opinions exist [27,28]. Hydrophilic preparations are intended to cause diffusion of fluids through the wound tissue and may help to clear surface wound debris. Copolymer flakes (Avalon; Summit Hill Lab, Navesink, New Jersey) enhance wound healing according to level 5 grade D expert opinion [27,28]. Dextranomer hydrophilic beads (Debrisan; Johnson & Johnson Products, New Brunswick, New Jersey) are reported to attract polymorphonuclear and mononuclear cells and may help to reduce excessive inflammation at the wound site [27,28].

Live Yeast-Cell Derivative

Live yeast-cell derivative (Preparation-H; Whitehall Lab, New York, New York) may stimulate oxygen consumption, epithelialization, and collagen synthesis in wounds. One researcher providing a level 5 grade D expert opinion states in several articles that he believed it did enhance epithelialization in dogs [27,28,47].

Petrolatum

One expert providing a level 5 grade D opinion states in several papers that petrolatum can adversely affect epithelialization [27] but can enhance wound contraction at 7 days [38]. Petrolatum and gauze 4 × 4 sponges can be used with petrolatum applied to the surface to create a nonadherent gauze type of wound dressing that may be more economically feasible compared with commercially available products.

Aloe Vera

Aloe vera has antiprostaglandin and antithromboxane properties that may reduce inflammation associated with wound healing. Because inflammation is a key component of healing, it should not be significantly reduced. Substances from the gel portion inside the aloe vera leaf can stimulate fibroblast replication in guinea pigs [48]. A level 5 grade D expert opinion does not recommend use of aloe vera on full-thickness wounds, in which inflammation is a key component of wound healing [28,31,47]. In pad wounds, aloe vera extract gel (Dermal wound gel) enhanced wound healing at 7 days compared with BNP and control groups. The gel also contains acemannan and allantoin; therefore, any or all of the components of the gel could be the actual cause of enhancement of wound healing.

Acemannan

Acemannan is a complex polymer containing mannose, and it is reported to enhance wound healing [28]. Two expert opinions recommend topical use of acemannan in several level 5 grade D reports [33–35]. It is available in a gel or freeze-dried form (Carravet Wound Dressing or Carra Sorb M; Carrington Laboratories, Irving, Texas).

Allantoin

Allantoin is reported to stimulate epithelial growth and tissue repair, especially in suppurative or chronic wounds [31]. Expert opinion in level 5 grade D studies recommends its use to enhance wound healing [33–35].

Maltodextrin NF

Maltodextrin NF is a D-glucose polysaccharide hydrophilic powder that reportedly yields glucose to provide energy for cell metabolism to enhance healing [35]. It has been reported to cause chemotaxis of polymorphonuclear cells, lymphocytes, and macrophages into wounds [35]. Maltodextrin NF (Intracell; Techni-Vet, Albuquerque, New Mexico) is recommended by one expert in two level 5 grade D reports [35].

Multipeptide Copper Complex

Tripeptide copper complex (TCC) is reported to cause chemoattraction of mast cells in vitro [49]. It also has a stimulating effect on cultured fibroblasts, resulting in increased collagen synthesis. In one level 1b grade A study in dogs, tripeptide copper and tetrapeptide copper preparations (PC 1020 and 1086; ProCyte Corporation, Kirkland, Washington) resulted in greater wound contraction and total healing at 7 days [49]. Both preparations can cause exuberant granulation tissue formation that may inhibit re-epithelialization [49]. In a level 1b grade A study of canine open pad wounds [31], TCC and acemannan (immunostimulant) were compared with respect to their effect on wound collagen content. The collagen content was measured objectively by use of hydroxyproline tissue content and special stains to identify collagen type. The use of TCC resulted in greater type I (mature) collagen, and the use of TCC and acemannan both resulted in more collagen than in a saline control group [31]. Level 5 grade B evidence recommending the use of TCC also exists [33–35]. Currently, products like Iamin Gel (ProCyte Corporation), containing copper peptide and hydrogel, are available.

SUMMARY

The authors commend the researchers who have reported the referenced publications with the limited financial and patient research resources available in veterinary medicine. The current state of veterinary literature regarding topical agents and their effect on wound granulation and epithelialization does not facilitate implementation of evidence-based medicine techniques. To the authors' knowledge, there are no published systematic reviews of randomized controlled trials. Although some randomized studies exist, they resemble a cohort study more closely than a controlled clinical trial. Cohort studies would be assigned a level 2 grade B status. For all randomized studies identified, there were no reports demonstrating repeatable results in the literature. Many of the randomized studies identified used quantitative measures, such as hand tracing followed by digitizing and planimetry, which is presumed to be less accurate than the more recently reported objective measures, such as digital photography, tissue hydroxyproline content, and LDPI.

Based on the literature identified in the authors' review, there is insufficient evidence to make a recommendation for or against any of the topical wound agents or procedures studied.

References

[1] Johnston DE. Wound healing in skin. Vet Clin North Am 1990;20(1):1–25.
[2] Pavletic M. Basic principles of wound healing. In: Pavletic M, editor. Atlas of small animal reconstructive surgery. Philadelphia: J.B. Lippincott; 1993. p. 11–8.
[3] Noli C, Miolo A. The mast cell in wound healing [review]. Vet Dermatol 2001;12:303–13.
[4] Hosgood G. Wound healing: the role of platelet-derived growth factor and transforming growth factor beta. Vet Surg 1993;22(6):490–5.
[5] Theoret CL. Growth factors in cutaneous wound repair. Compendium on Continuing Education for the Practicing Veterinarian 2001;23(4):383–9.
[6] Bohling MW, Henderson RA, Swaim SF, et al. Comparison of the role of the subcutaneous tissues in cutaneous wound healing in the dog and cat. Vet Surg 2006;35:3–14.
[7] Morgan PW, Binnington AG, Miller CW, et al. The effect of occlusive and semi-occlusive dressings on the healing of acute full-thickness skin wounds on the forelimbs of dogs. Vet Surg 1994;23:494–502.
[8] Swaim SF, Gillette RL, Sartin EA, et al. Effects of a hydrolyzed collagen dressing on the healing of open wounds in dogs. Am J Vet Res 2000;61(12):1574–8.
[9] Scardino MS, Swaim SF, Sartin EA, et al. Evaluation of treatment with a pulsed electromagnetic field on wound healing, clinicopathologic variables, and central nervous system activity of dogs. Am J Vet Res 1998;59(9):1177–81.
[10] Ramsey DT, Pope ER, Wagner-Mann C, et al. Effects of three occlusive dressing materials on healing of full-thickness skin wounds in dogs. Am J Vet Res 1995;56(7):941–9.
[11] Lee AH, Swaim SF, Yang ST, et al. Effects of gentamicin solution and cream on the healing of open wounds. Am J Vet Res 1984;45(8):1487–92.
[12] Vermeulen H, Ubbink D, Goossens A, et al. Dressings and topical agents for surgical wounds healing by secondary intention. Cochrane Database Syst Rev 2006;1464–780X:2. Available at: http://www.cochrane.org/reviews/en/ab003554.html. Accessed March 21, 2006.
[13] Smith-Akin KA, Bearden CF, Pittenger ST, et al. Toward a veterinary informatics research agenda: an analysis of the PubMed-indexed literature. Int J Med Inform 2007;76(4):306–12.
[14] Sanchez IR, Swaim SF, Nusbaum KE, et al. Effects of chlorhexidine diacetate and povidone-iodine on wound healing in dogs. Vet Surg 1988;17(6):291–5.
[15] Lineaweaver W, Howard R, Soucy D, et al. Topical antimicrobial toxicity. Arch Surg 1985;120:267–70.
[16] Lozier S, Pope E, Berg J. Effects of four preparations of 0.05% chlorhexidine diacetate on wound healing in dogs. Vet Surg 1992;21(2):107–12.
[17] Buffa EA, Lubbe AM, Verstraete FJM, et al. The effects of wound lavage solutions on canine fibroblasts: an in vitro study. Vet Surg 1997;26:460–6.
[18] Bohling MW, Henderson RA, Swaim SF, et al. Cutaneous wound healing in the cat: a microscopic description and comparison with cutaneous wound healing in the dog. Vet Surg 2004;33:579–87.

[19] Winkler JT, Swaim SF, Sartin EA, et al. The effect of porcine-derived small intestinal submucosa product on wounds with exposed bone in dogs. Vet Surg 2002;31:541–51.

[20] Swaim SF, Vaughn DM, Kincaid SA, et al. Effects of locally injected medications on healing of pad wounds in dogs. Am J Vet Res 1996;57(3):394–9.

[21] Available at: www.vin.com. Accessed April 2006.

[22] Phillps B, Ball C, Sackett D, et al. Available at: www.cebm.net/levels_of_evidence.asp. Accessed April 2006.

[23] Available at: http://library.downstate.edu/ebmdos/3toc.htm. Accessed April 2006.

[24] Olivry T, Mueller RS. Evidence-based veterinary dermatology: a systematic review of the pharmacotherapy of canine atopic dermatitis. Vet Dermatol 2003;14:121–46.

[25] Anonymous. Task force ratings. In: US Preventive Services Task Force, editor. Guide to clinical preventive services. 2nd edition. Washington, DC: U.S. Department of Health and Human Services; Office of Public Health and Science; Office of Disease Prevention and Health Promotion; 1996. p. 861–2.

[26] Sanchez IR, Nusbaum KE, Swaim SF, et al. Chlorhexidine diacetate and povidone-iodine cytotoxicity to canine embryonic fibroblasts and Staphylococcus aureus. Vet Surg 1988;17:182–5.

[27] Swaim SF. Bandages and topical agents. Vet Clin North Am Small Anim Pract 1990;20(1): 47–65.

[28] Swaim SF. Topical wound medications: a review. J Am Vet Med Assoc 1987;190(12): 1588–93.

[29] Rochat MC. Basic wound care and treatment. Vet Med April 2001;299–307.

[30] Liptak JM. An overview of the topical management of wounds. Aust Vet J 1997;75:408–13.

[31] Swaim SF, Riddell KP, McGuire JA. Effects of topical medications on the healing of open pad wounds in dogs. J Am Anim Hosp Assoc 1992;28:499–502.

[32] Bidlack DE. Furazolium chloride in management of skin infections and wounds of small animals and horses. Vet Med Small Anim Clin Nov 1967;1070–2.

[33] Zbigniew A, Wojciech B. Burn wounds management with occlusive dressing Granuflex IB in dogs. Presented at the WSAVA Proceedings. Granada, October 3–6, 2002.

[34] Swaim SF, Hinkle SH, Bradley DM. Wound contraction: basic and clinical factors. Comp Cont Ed 2001;23(1):20–34.

[35] Swaim SF, Gillette RL. An update on wound medications and dressings. Comp Cont Ed 1998;20(10):1133–46.

[36] Lee AH, Swaim SF, McGuire JA, et al. Effects of nonadherent dressing materials on the healing of open wounds in dogs. J Am Vet Med Assoc 1987;190(4):416–22.

[37] Holt TL, Mann FA. Carbon dioxide laser resection of a distal carpal pilomatricoma and wound closure using swine intestinal submucosa in a dog. J Am Anim Hosp Assoc 2003;39(5):499–505.

[38] Swaim SF. Wound management offers new alternatives. DVM Best Practices Feb 2002;4–6.

[39] Ueno H, Yamada H, Tanaka I, et al. Accelerating effects of chitosan for healing at early phase of experimental open wound in dogs. Biomaterials 1999;20:1407–14.

[40] Ueno H, Mori T, Fujinaga T. Topical formulations and wound healing applications of chitosan. Adv Drug Deliv Rev 2001;52(2):105–15.

[41] Okamoto Y, Shibazaki K, Minami S, et al. Evaluation of chitin and chitosan on open wound healing in dogs. J Vet Med Sci 1995;57(5):851–4.

[42] Lucroy MD, Edwards BJ, Madewell BR. Low-intensity laser light-induced closure of a chronic wound in a dog. Vet Surg 1999;28:292–5.

[43] Tanaka A, Nagate T, Matsuda H. Acceleration of wound healing by gelatin film dressings in epidermal growth factor. J Vet Med Sci 2005;67(9):909–13.

[44] Eisinger M, Sadan S, Soehnchen R, et al. Wound healing by epidermal-derived factors: experimental and preliminary clinical studies. Prog Clin Biol Res 1988;266:291–302.

[45] Mathews KA, Binnington AG. Wound management using sugar. Comp Cont Ed 2002; 24(1):41–50.

[46] Mathews KA, Binnington AG. Wound management using honey. Comp Cont Ed 2002; 24(1):53–60.
[47] Fitch RB, Swaim SF. The role of epithelialization in wound healing. Comp Cont Ed 1995; 17(2):167–77.
[48] Rodriguez-Bigas M, Cruz NI, Suarez A. Comparative evaluation of aloe vera in the management of burn wounds in guinea pigs. Plast Reconstr Surg 1988;81:386–9.
[49] Swaim SF, Bradley DM, Spano JS, et al. Evaluation of multipeptide-copper complex medications on open wound healing in dogs. J Am Anim Hosp Assoc 1993;29:519–25.

Vet Clin Small Anim 37 (2007) 579–609

VETERINARY CLINICS
SMALL ANIMAL PRACTICE

Thromboembolic Therapies in Dogs and Cats: An Evidence-Based Approach

Kari V. Lunsford, DVM*,
Andrew J. Mackin, MVS, DVSc

Department of Clinical Sciences, College of Veterinary Medicine, Mail Stop 9825, Spring Street, Mississippi State University, Mississippi State, MS 39762–6100, USA

EVIDENCE-BASED MEDICINE

The goal of evidence-based medicine is to use the best evidence from clinical research in combination with clinical expertise and patient and client factors in guiding the care of individual patients. Detailed guidelines for the evaluation of research evidence and clinical recommendations related to therapy of thromboembolic disease in human patients have been reviewed [1,2]. These guidelines call for data originating from large, well-designed, randomized controlled clinical trials evaluating therapies in clearly defined patient populations with naturally occurring diseases without comorbidity [3]. This approach cannot be practically applied to the veterinary literature, however, because the criteria would eliminate most of the available veterinary literature from the "best evidence" pool and few, if any, strong treatment recommendations could be made. In veterinary medicine, we are therefore forced to make use of less ideal "evidence," such as extrapolation from experimental studies in dogs and cats without naturally occurring diseases and from clinical trials in other species (particularly human clinical trials), as well as limited information gained from veterinary clinical experience, small clinical trials, case studies, and anecdotal reports. In this article, although specific treatment recommendations have been made for each of the common thromboembolic conditions seen in dogs and cats, these recommendations are made with the important caveat that, to date, such suggested therapeutic approaches are based on limited evidence.

THROMBOEMBOLIC THERAPIES

Medical treatment aimed at thromboembolic diseases consists of dissolving existing thrombi (thrombolytic drugs) or preventing new thrombus formation, primarily by means of the use of antiplatelet drugs, heparin products, and vitamin K antagonists. Each of these specific drug classes is briefly reviewed

*Corresponding author. E-mail address: lunsford@cvm.msstate.edu (K.V. Lunsford).

0195-5616/07/$ – see front matter
doi:10.1016/j.cvsm.2007.01.010

separately, and a coordinated approach to treating existing thrombi and preventing thrombus formation in the first place is then discussed.

THROMBOLYTIC DRUG OVERVIEW

Thrombolytic therapies are targeted toward existing thrombi. Current therapies in human medicine include systemic thrombolytic drugs, local thrombolytic drugs, and mechanical or surgical extraction. Systemic and local drugs include streptokinase (Kabikinase, Streptase); urokinase (Abbokinase); and recombinant tissue plasminogen activator (rt-PA) agents, such as alteplase (Activase), reteplase (Retavase), and tenecteplase (TNKase).

The rt-PA products activate plasminogen to form plasmin, which degrades fibrin, resulting in clot lysis. Circulating plasminogen binds to fibrin formed at sites of vascular injury and clot formation. The rt-PA products activate bound plasminogen much more rapidly than they activate freely circulating plasminogen; thus, these products are described as "clot-specific" agents. At pharmacologic concentrations, however, a systemic lytic state can occur, creating a considerable risk for bleeding [4].

Streptokinase is produced by β-hemolytic streptococci. Streptokinase forms stable complexes with plasminogen, inducing a conformational change that promotes the formation of plasmin. Streptokinase is not fibrin dependent and readily binds free circulating plasminogen, leading to a systemic lytic state. Preformed antibodies to streptokinase may exist secondary to previous streptococcal infections; therefore, loading doses are recommended to overcome antibody inactivation. Urokinase is a protease that is produced by kidney cells and is naturally found in urine. Like streptokinase, urokinase is fibrin independent and binds circulating plasminogen, leading to a systemic lytic state [4].

ANTIPLATELET DRUG OVERVIEW

Traditionally, antiplatelet therapy in people has consisted of low-dose aspirin, although, more recently, newer agents, such as ticlopidine (Ticlid) and clopidogrel (Plavix) have also been used.

Aspirin irreversibly inhibits the cyclooxygenase (COX) activities of PGH synthase-1 and PGH synthase-2 (COX-1 and COX-2) [5]. These enzymes catalyze the conversion of arachidonic acid to PGH_2, the precursor for PGD_2, PGE_2, $PGE_{2\alpha}$, PGI_2, and thromboxane A_2 (TXA_2). Platelets primarily process PGH_2 to TXA_2, whereas vascular endothelial cells primarily process PGH_2 to prostacyclin (PGI_2). TXA_2 enhances platelet function and primary hemostasis by inducing platelet aggregation and vasoconstriction, whereas PGI_2 inhibits hemostasis by impeding platelet aggregation and inducing vasodilation [6]. TXA_2 is produced by platelets by means of the actions of COX-1 in response to short-term cytokine signals, whereas PGI_2 is produced by the vasculature by means of the actions of COX-2 as well as COX-1 [7,8]. In human beings, aspirin is 50 to 100 times more potent against platelet-derived COX-1 than against monocyte or endothelial cell–derived COX-2 [9]. Furthermore, aspirin produces a permanent defect in platelet TXA_2 synthesis, because platelets lack a nucleus, and thus cannot produce more active COX-1 enzyme, whereas inhibition of PGI_2 production by nucleated vascular endothelial cells is temporary. Platelet function is therefore extremely sensitive to inhibition by aspirin, and the drug produces an antithrombotic state over a wide range of doses [9–12]. In people, once-daily low-dose aspirin is sufficient to maintain complete inhibition of TXA_2 synthesis, whereas inhibition of PGI_2 synthesis requires much higher and more frequent aspirin doses. Careful aspirin dosing can thus impair platelet function without significantly reducing the beneficial antithrombotic effects of PGI_2.

Aspirin pharmacodynamics in people, dogs, and cats are similar, and dogs have served as an animal model for many preclinical studies of the antiplatelet effects of aspirin. Feline aspirin pharmacokinetics, in contrast, are different because of a relative deficiency of glucuronate in cats. Aspirin has a prolonged elimination half-life of approximately 38 hours in the cat compared with 15 to 20 minutes in people and approximately 7 hours in dogs.

Ticlopidine and clopidogrel are thienopyridines that selectively inhibit ADP-induced platelet aggregation but have no direct effects on arachidonic acid metabolism [13]. Neither drug has an effect on ADP-induced platelet aggregation in vitro, suggesting that hepatic biotransformation is needed to produce an active metabolite. The clinical effects and pharmacodynamics of clopidogrel have been evaluated in cats, and significant antiplatelet effects can be achieved in this species [14].

HEPARIN OVERVIEW

Standard available heparin products include unfractionated heparin (UFH) and low-molecular-weight heparin (LMWH), such as enoxaparin (Lovenox) and dalteparin (Fragmin).

UFH is a mixture of glycosaminoglycan molecules with variable sizes, anticoagulant activities, and pharmacokinetic properties [15]. The molecular weight of UFH ranges from 3000 to 30,000 d, with a mean of 15,000 d (approximately 45 monosaccharide units) [16]. Heparin complexes with and catalyzes the activity of the anticoagulant protein antithrombin. The heparin:antithrombin complex inhibits coagulation factors IIa (thrombin), IXa, Xa, Xia, and XIIa. Only approximately one third of UFH molecules contain the binding site for antithrombin, and the remaining two thirds have minimal anticoagulant activity [17]. The clotting factors thrombin and factor Xa are most sensitive to the activities of the heparin:antithrombin complex. Only heparin molecules that contain more than 18 monosaccharide units are capable of inactivating thrombin, although smaller heparin molecules can successfully bind and inactivate factor Xa in the presence of antithrombin [18]. By inactivating thrombin, heparin not only prevents fibrin formation but inhibits thrombin-induced platelet activation and continued activation of coagulation factors V and VIII [19–21]. The biologic effects of UFH and other heparin products are quite variable and depend on the proportion of heparin molecules large enough to bind thrombin.

The pharmacokinetics of UFH are unpredictable as well. Larger heparin molecules are cleared from the circulation relatively rapidly because of binding to plasma proteins, macrophages, and endothelial cells, which is a saturable process. Remaining smaller heparin molecules, those with a lower ratio of anti-IIa to anti-Xa activity, are cleared more slowly by renal mechanisms [15]. Because of this high degree of variability in pharmacokinetics and biologic activity, UFH therapy must be monitored closely and titrated to effect to avoid undertreatment or bleeding complications. The test that is routinely used to measure UFH effect is the activated partial thromboplastin time (aPTT), with an accepted therapeutic target range of 1.5 to 2.5 times the normal control aPTT value. The pharmacokinetic properties of UFH in dogs are similar to those in people [22].

LMWH is derived from UFH by chemical or enzymatic depolymerization and has been developed in response to some of the difficulties associated with UFH therapy. LMWH has a mean molecular weight of 4000 to 5,000 d (approximately one third that of UFH), comprising roughly 15 monosaccharide units per molecule. In general, LMWH has reduced anti-IIa activity relative to anti-Xa activity and also has better pharmacokinetic properties.

LMWH fractions have progressively smaller effects on factor IIa (thrombin) activity, because the mean molecular weight of the fraction decreases. LMWH, like UFH, binds to and catalyzes the activity of antithrombin; however, only 25% to 50% of the heparin molecules in LMWH are large enough to inhibit factor IIa, although all retain the capacity to inactivate factor Xa. UFH has an anti-Xa/anti-IIa ratio of 1:1, whereas LMWH preparations have ratios ranging from 2:1 to 4:1 [15]. Compared with UFH, LMWH at standard doses has a minimal effect on aPTT, because the prolonged aPTT seen with UFH therapy primarily reflects inhibition of factor IIa. Inhibition of factor Xa, in contrast, has little effect on aPTT [23].

The available LMWH preparations are variable in their pharmacokinetic profiles and are not clinically interchangeable [15]. LMWH has a reduced affinity for binding to plasma proteins or cells compared with UFH, leading to a more predictable dose response relation and longer half-life, because most of the LMWH molecules undergo renal clearance [24]. LMWH preparations have a bioavailability after subcutaneous administration of nearly 100% at low doses, and peak activity consistently occurs between 3 and 5 hours after administration [25]. The predictability of LMWH pharmacokinetics in people allows administration at a fixed dose without routine monitoring of therapeutic efficacy. Few pharmacokinetic studies have been performed in special human patient populations, such as those with renal failure or morbid obesity, and monitoring is therefore suggested in these patients [26]. Chromogenic assays of anti-factor Xa activity are the recommended laboratory method for monitoring LMWH therapy, although the relation between clinical effect and anti-Xa activity is not entirely clear. Anti-factor Xa levels are inversely related to propagation of existing thrombi and development of new thrombi, although the minimum effective level of Xa activity inhibition has not been ascertained with certainty [15,27]. The pharmacokinetics of LMWH in dogs have been evaluated, and therapeutic anti-factor Xa levels can be achieved [28,29].

VITAMIN K ANTAGONIST OVERVIEW

The vitamin K antagonists have played an important role in the management of thromboembolic disease in people for more than 50 years. The use of vitamin K antagonists is not without considerable challenge, however, because these drugs have narrow therapeutic windows and considerable interindividual variability in dose response relation, are prone to many dietary and drug interactions, have monitoring assays that are difficult to standardize, and are prone to problems with patient compliance [30].

Warfarin (Coumadin), the most commonly used therapeutic vitamin K antagonist worldwide, interferes with the cyclic interconversion of vitamin K and vitamin K oxide, thus impairing the hepatic carboxylation of the vitamin K–dependent coagulation factors II, VII, IX, and X [31,32]. Because these clotting factors require carboxylation to become activated, exposure to warfarin leads to the hepatic production of decarboxylated proteins with greatly reduced coagulant activity [33–35]. Warfarin similarly inhibits the anticoagulant factors protein C and protein S. Because protein C has a circulating half-life that is shorter than that of most of the clotting factors, warfarin has the potential to create a transient procoagulant state before anticoagulant effects are maximized. Heparinization is therefore recommended at the onset of warfarin therapy for most patients [30]. The anticoagulant effects of warfarin can be overcome with low doses of vitamin K_1, and large doses of the vitamin can lead to warfarin resistance for up to 1 week or more [33].

Warfarin is rapidly absorbed after oral administration and reaches peak blood levels approximately 90 minutes later, with a half-life of 36 to 42 hours in human beings [36]. Warfarin circulates bound to plasma proteins (primarily albumin) before being accumulated in the liver [30]. Diet, concurrent drug administration, and disease states can all potentially affect the pharmacokinetics of warfarin. Because of the drug's unpredictable pharmacokinetics, therapeutic drug monitoring is essential for all patients receiving warfarin. The prothrombin time (PT) is used to monitor warfarin therapy and is sensitive to significant reductions in levels of factors II, VII, and X. Measurement of PT is performed by adding calcium and thromboplastin to citrated plasma. Thromboplastin from differing sources can vary considerably in biologic activity, and can therefore lead to inconsistent PT results. The activity of thromboplastin is described by the International Sensitivity Index (ISI), which is a comparison of any given thromboplastin with primary World Health Organization (WHO) international reference preparations; the lower the ISI, the more active is the thromboplastin [30]. In 1982, a model for standardizing PT results based on the ISI of the thromboplastin used [37] was adopted, in which the laboratory PT result is converted into the international normalization ratio (INR = [Patient PT/Mean Normal PT]ISI). This standardization method has not been well validated in dogs and cats.

THROMBOLYTIC THERAPIES

Thrombolytic Therapy in People

Thromboembolic diseases can, for the sake of this discussion, be classified as those affecting primarily the arterial circulation, such as arterial thrombosis or embolism; those affecting primarily the venous circulation, such as deep vein thrombosis; and those affecting both, as in pulmonary thromboembolism (PTE). Thromboembolic disease associated with the venous circulation, although associated with considerable morbidity, is rarely life threatening on its own, whereas acute arterial thromboembolic episodes or pulmonary thromboembolic episodes can result in sudden death. These considerations are important when discussing thrombolytic therapies.

The leading causes for acute arterial occlusion in people are thrombosis, embolism, and trauma [38]. Trauma is typically associated with arterial laceration, transection, and external compressive forces (fractures or luxations). Iatrogenic trauma in association with diagnostic and therapeutic catheter placement is also a relatively common cause of vascular occlusion. Treatment in otherwise healthy vessels typically consists of surgery or ballooning to re-establish vascular patency, followed by short-term anticoagulant therapy with UFH if there are no risk factors for bleeding complications.

Nontraumatic arterial thrombi are often associated with cardiac valvular disease, prosthetic valves, and atrial fibrillation but may also be associated with atherosclerosis, aneurysms, recent endovascular procedures, and venous thrombosis. Advanced atherosclerotic disease is the most common cause of arterial thrombosis in human patients [38]. Surgical embolectomy is the preferred therapy whenever possible in the case of acute occlusion of healthy peripheral arteries. Balloon catheterization and percutaneous thromboembolectomy procedures have recently been used as alternatives to open surgical procedures; however, there have been no randomized comparisons of the procedures [38].

Thrombolytic drugs, such as streptokinase, urokinase, and tissue plasminogen activator (t-PA), provide a therapeutic alternative to surgical restoration of circulation. The systemic application of thrombolytic agents by intravenous infusion has been largely replaced by catheter-directed local administration of drugs at the site of arterial thrombus formation. Currently, the rt-PA drugs are the most widely used thrombolytics, and several new rt-PA preparations are under investigation for use as primary thrombolytics [39,40].

In direct comparisons in naturally occurring disease in human patients with arterial thromboembolic disease, rt-PA administered intra-arterially by means of a catheter was superior when compared with intra-arterial streptokinase and systemic intravenous rt-PA, with 30-day limb salvage rates of 80%, 60%, and 45%, respectively [41]. Another study, also in naturally occurring human disease, demonstrated faster early clot lysis with rt-PA than with urokinase, although the 24-hour lysis rate and 30-day clinical success rate were similar with the two drugs [42]. Other studies in people comparing urokinase with rt-PA resulted in similar findings [43,44].

Two meta-analyses compared the mortality and amputation rates in human patients with acute limb ischemia undergoing thrombolytic therapy or surgical vascular restoration and found the rates to be similar, although bleeding and distal embolization occurred more frequently with thrombolytic therapy [45,46]. Although many other studies [47–52] have also compared surgical thrombectomy with medical thrombolysis in people, there is no clear-cut evidence supporting one intervention over the other in patients with nontraumatic arterial occlusion. One recent recommendation is that intra-arterial thrombolytic therapy rather than surgical embolectomy be performed in human patients in the acute (<14 days) phase of arterial thrombosis if there is a low risk of myonecrosis and ischemic neuropathy developing during the time it takes for revascularization to occur [38].

Unlike arterial thrombi, which are typically associated with an acute risk of ischemia and serious organ or tissue damage, venous thrombi often do not present an immediate danger to affected tissues, and emergency medical thrombolysis of venous thrombi is thus often not indicated. In fact, there is no clear evidence in the human literature supporting the early lysis of venous thrombi, especially considering that it is well established that thrombolytic therapies significantly increase the risk for bleeding. Conservative management with anticoagulants alone, without concurrent thrombolysis, does not seem to increase the risk for death or recurrence of the thrombus [53]. An overview of randomized trials comparing intravenous streptokinase thrombolysis with conservative heparin anticoagulant therapy in human patients with deep vein thrombosis revealed that although complete thrombolysis was achieved more frequently in patients treated with streptokinase, treated individuals were nearly three times more prone to bleeding [54]. Comparable studies using urokinase and rt-PA as thrombolytic agents demonstrated similar results [55]. Because of the high incidence of bleeding complications, the routine use of thrombolytic therapy in people with deep vein thrombosis is therefore not advised, except in those patients at immediate risk for loss of a limb [53].

Because PTE is more likely than venous thrombosis to be immediately life threatening, it would intuitively be expected that thrombolytic therapy might be indicated in patients with PTE. Various thrombolytic agents have been assessed in human patients with PTE, and streptokinase, urokinase, and rt-PA have all been shown to have similar efficacy when comparing posttreatment angiographic changes and improvement in pulmonary vascular resistances, although rt-PA requires a much shorter (2 hours) infusion time than urokinase (12 hours) or streptokinase (24 hours) [56–59]. Although thrombolytic therapy in people with PTE leads to more rapid resolution of radiographic and hemodynamic changes than does anticoagulant therapy alone, there is no difference in the resolution of symptoms or in the mortality rate between the two treatment modalities [60]. In fact, there is no clear evidence supporting thrombolytic therapy for human patients with acute PTE. Several studies [61–65] have shown that the mortality rates attributable to PTE in people are as low as 2% when the condition is promptly diagnosed and treated with appropriate anticoagulant therapy alone. Concurrent treatment of such patients with thrombolytics increases the risk of intracranial bleeding, a potentially life-threatening complication of therapy, to approximately 1% to 2% [66]. Systemic thrombolytic drugs are therefore not routinely recommended for the treatment of PTE in people, except in those patients with massive PTE who are hemodynamically unstable. Local administration of thrombolytic drugs for treatment of PTE is also not recommended in people, and when thrombolysis is indicated, systemic agents with shorter infusion times are preferred.

Thrombolytic Therapy in Small Animals

Dogs and cats have been used as experimental models for human disease in countless preclinical studies evaluating thrombolytic drugs and surgical procedures; however, there is little information regarding thrombolytic therapy in naturally occurring small animal diseases. In fact, a recent review of thrombolytics in veterinary medicine concluded that because of the small number of animals with naturally occurring diseases treated and the relative lack of associated data, it was impossible to make specific recommendations with regard to thrombolytic therapy [67]. In particular, there is limited information available to permit solid evidence-based evaluation of the use of thrombolytic therapy in the two conditions in which such therapy is most likely to be considered in small animal medicine: arterial thrombosis (particularly arterial thromboembolism [ATE] in cats) and PTE in dogs.

The thrombolytics streptokinase and rt-PA have been evaluated, at least to a limited extent, in cats and dogs with ATE. A 1986 study [68] evaluating the use of streptokinase in experimental ATE in cats established that a loading dose of 90,000 IU given intravenously over 20 to 30 minutes followed by an infusion of 45,000 IU per hour reliably induced a systemic fibrinolytic state but failed to produce clinical improvement or a significant reduction in clot size at necropsy. In a 1996 case series [69] describing the use of streptokinase in 8 cats with naturally occurring ATE or left atrial thrombi, all cats unfortunately died during treatment. In a more recent retrospective study [59] describing the use of streptokinase in 46 cats with ATE, although 25 patients achieved return of femoral pulses within a day of commencing therapy, 18 affected cats died in the hospital and an additional 13 were euthanized because of poor response to therapy or treatment complications. A 1988 review [70] discussed the use of rt-PA in cats with naturally occurring ATE; although 50% of treated cats were reported to regain perfusion and use of limbs within 36 hours of initiating therapy, mortality rates were high (50%) and were attributed to reperfusion hyperkalemia during clot lysis. Interestingly, conservative therapy with aspirin alone in cats with naturally occurring ATE has been reported to be associated with a comparable 50% rate return of perfusion and limb function [71], and there is thus no clear evidence supporting the use of thrombolytics in cats with ATE. In dogs, a 1996 study [72] described the successful use of streptokinase in 4 patients treated for naturally occurring ATE, and a more recent case report describes the successful use of streptokinase and dalteparin in another young dog with ATE [73]. There is also a single case report from 1998 [74] describing the successful use of the rt-PA alteplase for the dissolution of a distal aortic thrombus in a dog. Apart from a single case report in 2002 describing the successful use of catheter assisted rt-PA administration in a dog with thrombosis of the cranial vena cava [75], there have been no clinical reports on the use of thrombolytics for small animals with venous thrombosis, and there have also been no clinical studies evaluating the use of thrombolytic therapy in naturally occurring PTE in dogs or cats.

Recommendations for Thrombolytic Therapy in Small Animals

- Thrombolytic therapy should not be used in the management of ATE in cats.
- Thrombolytic therapy may reduce morbidity and mortality in some cases of ATE in dogs.
- No specific recommendations can be made based on the available veterinary literature with regard to thrombolytic agents in venous thrombosis or PTE.
- Based on extrapolation from the human literature, however, the use thrombolytic therapy is not indicated for most patients with venous thrombosis or PTE.
- Thrombolytic therapy may be indicated in veterinary patients with hemodynamically unstable acute PTE or with venous thrombosis associated with severe or unacceptable morbidity.
- If thrombolytic therapy is to be performed, agents requiring shorter infusion times, such as rt-PA, may be preferred. Alteplase has been used in dogs at a dose of 1 mg/kg given as an intravenous bolus every 60 minutes for a total of 10 doses concurrently with an infusion of lactated Ringer's solution at a rate of 9 mL/h. The cost of one 50-mg vial of alteplase, however, is approximately $1700.

MAINTENANCE THERAPIES

Maintenance Therapy in People

Long-term thrombotic conditions in people tend to be treated with anticoagulant drugs that prevent further thrombus formation rather than with thrombolytic agents. Even in conditions that may require initial thrombolysis or embolectomy, such as acute arterial emboli or thrombosis, it is typically recommended that immediate systemic anticoagulation with UFH be commenced to prevent thrombotic propagation and that anticoagulation then be continued with long-term vitamin K antagonists [38]. There are, however, no formal studies establishing the unequivocal benefit of any anticoagulant agent in this role in the treatment of human patients with acute arterial embolic diseases.

Anticoagulation is the mainstay of the early management of deep vein thromboses in people. The goal is to prevent thrombus propagation and early recurrence as well as to reduce the incidence of PTE, a serious complication of venous thrombi. Patients are typically started on anticoagulant therapy as soon as possible; in fact, if there is a delay in objective diagnosis and clinical suspicion is high, treatment is commenced before confirming the diagnosis. Initial therapy for venous thrombosis consists of heparinization with subcutaneous LMWH, intravenous UFH, or subcutaneous UFH. Short-term therapy with UFH followed by a long-term vitamin K antagonist, such as warfarin, has been shown to be as effective as long-term UFH therapy [76]. The current recommendation in people is to begin heparin and vitamin K antagonists simultaneously, stopping the heparin therapy 5 to 7 days after the INR has stabilized [77]. The use of warfarin alone is not recommended because of the risk of an early prothrombotic phase associated with protein C deficiency [78].

For a long time, intravenous UFH was the heparinization method of choice for the initial management of deep vein thromboses in people. The biologic effect of UFH, however, is unpredictable on an intra- and interpatient basis. Additionally, UFH has a narrow therapeutic window, and thus requires close monitoring during the initial stages of treatment, because a minimum level of anticoagulation must be maintained throughout the treatment period to ensure efficacy. The recommended dose of intravenous UFH (used concurrently with warfarin) for the initial management of deep vein thromboses in people is a bolus of 5000 U followed by a continuous infusion of 30,000 U for the first 24 hours or a weight-adjusted bolus of 80 U/kg followed by 18 U/kg/h for 24 hours. Subsequent UFH doses should then be adjusted according to aPTT monitoring [77]. Intermittent intravenous dosing of UFH is not recommended, because this protocol is associated with a greater risk of bleeding than is intravenous infusion [79].

Subcutaneous UFH every 12 hours can be used instead of intravenous UFH as long as careful monitoring is performed and dose adjustments are made to achieve therapeutic aPTT levels. Subcutaneous administration of UFH in people has been shown to be as safe and effective as continuous intravenous administration [80]. The recommended subcutaneous UFH protocol is an initial intravenous bolus of 5000 U followed by 17,500 U subcutaneously every 12 hours for the first day, with subsequent doses titrated to aPTT [77]. Subcutaneous UFH can be used when warfarin is not recommended, such as in patients with cancer [81], although UFH has largely been replaced by LMWH more recently.

Several studies have compared intravenous UFH and LMWH, used concurrently with warfarin, in the initial management of deep vein thromboses in people and have concluded that LMWH is equally as safe and effective and provides cost-saving benefits and improved quality of life because of the reduced need for monitoring and the possibility of at-home management [61,82,83]. Although most studies have evaluated twice-daily dosing protocols for LMWH, several studies have reported that once-daily dosing is equally as safe and effective in most patients [84,85]. At least three randomized clinical trials [76,86,87] have evaluated the use of LMWH for the long-term management of deep vein thromboses in people and have determined that treatment with subcutaneous LMWH is as effective as oral warfarin in most patients and is more effective in patients with cancer. Furthermore, there were fewer bleeding complications seen with LMWH compared with warfarin. LMWH allows weight-adjusted doses to be given once or twice daily, typically without monitoring. In certain circumstances, such as renal failure, however, the LMWH dose may need to be adjusted based on chromogenic anti-factor Xa assays. The recommended therapeutic range for anti-factor Xa activity is 0.6 to 1.0 IU/mL for twice-daily LMWH dosing, whereas higher anti-factor Xa activity (1.0–2.0 IU/mL) is acceptable for once-daily dosing [77].

There is clear evidence supporting the use of initial and long-term warfarin in human patients with deep vein thromboses. A 1985 study showed that patients who did not receive warfarin had a high rate of thrombus extension or recurrence in spite of initial treatment with intravenous UFH [88]. Another study evaluated subcutaneous low-dose UFH as an alternative to warfarin for long-term treatment of deep vein thrombosis and documented a high rate (almost 50%) of thrombus recurrence [89]. In people with deep vein thromboses, ongoing warfarin therapy should be adjusted to maintain an INR between 2.0 and 3.0 [90–93]. The optimal duration of therapy with warfarin depends on disease history and concurrent illness. A recent study has shown that continued elevation in plasma D-dimer levels after the discontinuation of warfarin is associated with an increased risk of recurrence of thrombosis [94]. Although warfarin is the preferred treatment for deep vein thrombosis in people, there are some instances when the drug may be contraindicated, such as during pregnancy or in patients with cancer [81]. In human patients with cancer who have deep vein thromboses, several studies have documented improved efficacy of LMWH compared with warfarin [76,86,87].

The treatment recommendations for the management of PTE in people are generally the same as the treatment recommendations for deep vein thromboses. Clinical trials have validated the efficacy of similar treatment regimens used in patients with deep vein thromboses alone, deep vein thromboses with PTE, and PTE alone [77].

Maintenance Therapy for Arterial Thromboembolism in Small Animals

Suggested therapies for established ATE in dogs and cats include dietary modification (n-3 fatty acids), aspirin, warfarin, heparin (UFH or LMWH), and, recently, the platelet inhibitor clopidogrel. Most veterinary recommendations for treating ATE come from anecdotal experience and limited experimental and clinical trials rather than from extrapolation from the human literature, because limited formal studies have been performed in people with comparable conditions.

Although increased dietary levels of n-3 fatty acids have been shown to decrease platelet function in some species, a 1994 study evaluated dietary n-3 fatty acid supplementation in normal cats and found no alteration in platelet function or bleeding time [95]. A similar study in dogs demonstrated that dietary n-6-to–n-3 ratios had no effect on hemostatic parameters [96].

Based on pathophysiologic rationale and clinical experience, aspirin therapy has been recommended as part of the initial management of feline ATE for many years at a dose of 81 mg per cat every 48 to 72 hours [97,98]. A recently published retrospective study comparing cats with ATE treated with "high-dose" (>40 mg per cat every 72 hours) and "low-dose" (5 mg per cat every 72 hour) aspirin found no difference in survival or recurrence rate between the two treatment groups, with more frequent and severe adverse reactions in the high-dose group, suggesting that if aspirin is to be used in cats, a low dose is preferable [99]. Aspirin therapy was reported in a 2000 case series of six dogs with ATE; the drug was used in the three dogs that survived the initial thrombotic episode, and in those dogs that survived for more than a month, there was no recurrence of clinical signs [100].

Warfarin has also been recommended for the treatment of ATE in cats at a dose of 0.25 to 0.5 mg/d per cat [101,102] or at a lower dose of 0.1 to 0.2 mg/d per cat [103]. Pharmacokinetic and pharmacodynamic studies in cats have demonstrated that a warfarin dose of 0.06 to 0.09 mg/kg/d is appropriate, although there is considerable intrapatient variability [104,105]. Difficulty arises in dosing warfarin in cats. Because the differently active warfarin enantiomers are not evenly distributed within tablets, warfarin tablets must be finely crushed and carefully compounded for precise dosing [104]. Additionally, frequent and costly monitoring of clotting is necessary to avoid bleeding complications. As a result of these difficulties, the use of aspirin is often preferred over the use of warfarin in the treatment and prevention of ATE in cats [106]. One small study evaluated the use of warfarin in the treatment of 17 cats with ATE compared with 14 cats treated with the LMWH dalteparin and reported that the warfarin group had a median survival time of 69 days and a 24% rate of re-embolism and that all the cats with a second embolic episode died [107]. Warfarin has also been advocated as an anticoagulant therapy for dogs at a dose of 0.1 to 0.2 mg/kg/d [101], but no studies have demonstrated the efficacy or benefit of this approach over other forms of anticoagulation.

A 2004 review of therapy for feline ATE provided recommendations based on author experience and expertise and suggested treatment with subcutaneous UFH at an initial dose of 250 to 300 U/kg every 8 hours [106]. Alternatively, based on clinical experience and unpublished data on the LMWH enoxaparin, the authors suggested an enoxaparin dose of 100 U/kg (1 mg/kg) given as often as every 8 hours [106]. A 2004 retrospective study evaluated another LMWH, dalteparin, in 57 cats with ATE and determined that it was easily administered and well tolerated in cats [108]. This study showed that 25% (5 of 20) of the cats with at least one previous ATE episode had a recurrence while receiving dalteparin. Another smaller study comparing dalteparin and warfarin, however, demonstrated a 43% rate of re-embolization in the dalteparin group [107]. For comparison, previous studies published ATE recurrence rates in cats ranging from 25% to 75% [59,99,109–111]. Pharmacokinetic studies in normal cats have shown that a single subcutaneous dose of dalteparin at a rate of 100 U/kg attains the desired therapeutic range of anti-factor Xa activity extrapolated from human data [108].

The antiplatelet effects and pharmacodynamics of clopidogrel were evaluated in five normal cats in 2004, and significant antiplatelet effects were seen at doses of 18.75 mg/d, 37.5 mg/d, and 75 mg/d, with no adverse effects [14]. An in vitro study of the effects of clopidogrel on rt-PA–induced thrombolysis of feline thrombi, however, showed that it had no effect on the rate of thrombolysis [112].

Recommendations for Maintenance Therapy for Arterial Thromboembolism in Small Animals

- Dietary supplementation with n-3 fatty acids is not recommended for the management of ATE in dogs or cats.

- Aspirin is recommended for feline ATE at a dose of 5 mg/kg administered every 72 hours.
- Warfarin can be considered in the management of cats with ATE at a dose of 0.6 to 0.9 mg/kg/d, although there are not sufficient studies documenting any benefit in using warfarin over other anticoagulant therapies. Heparinization is recommended during the first 5 to 7 days that warfarin is administered.
- Subcutaneous UFH should also be considered at a dose of 250 to 300 U/kg every 8 hours for the initial in-hospital therapy of feline ATE. Enoxaparin or dalteparin can be considered as an alternative to UFH. Both have been used at a dose of 100 U/kg (or 1 mg/kg for enoxaparin) given every 12 to 24 hours, although there are no clinical studies directly comparing the efficacies of any of the various methods of heparinization.
- Clopidogrel is not recommended as adjunct therapy for clot lysis. Clopidogrel, however, may eventually prove to be a reasonable alternative to aspirin for the management of feline ATE, although there are no studies evaluating its use in clinical patients.
- There is insufficient evidence to make a recommendation regarding aspirin therapy in dogs with ATE at this time.

Maintenance Therapy for Pulmonary Thromboembolism in Small Animals

There is little evidence pertaining to the management of deep vein thrombosis or PTE in the veterinary literature. Many recommendations are limited to the treatment of underlying conditions and supportive care, whereas anticoagulant recommendations are largely extrapolated from human therapies. Warfarin has been used in dogs and cats at starting doses of 0.22 mg/kg administered every 12 hours in dogs and 0.5 mg per cat administered once daily initially and then adjusted to achieve a PT prolongation of 1.25 to 1.5 times the pretreatment value [113]. One study evaluated loading doses of warfarin and INR values in dogs and concluded that two 6-mg doses of warfarin given 24 hours apart safely achieve an INR between 2.0 and 3.0 in dogs weighing 25 to 30 kg, although the utility of using the INR to titrate therapy in dogs has not been established [114]. This same study advocated initiating UFH concurrently with warfarin. In dogs, a constant rate infusion of UFH at a rate of 10 to 25 U/kg/h [115] or subcutaneous UFH at a dose of 200 to 500 U/kg every 8 hours adjusted to reach a target aPTT of 1.5 to 2 times the pretreatment values is recommended [116–118]. A recent study evaluating the use of an anti-factor Xa assay in dogs, however, suggests that this parameter may be more reliable than aPTT for the monitoring of UFH; the recommended canine therapeutic range for anti-factor Xa activity was 0.35 to 0.70 U/mL [119]. The recommended starting dose range of UFH is wide because of the unpredictable pharmacokinetics and biologic activity of subcutaneous UFH in dogs; anecdotal clinical experiences suggest that 200 U/kg undertreats most dogs, whereas 500 U/kg can be associated with a significantly increased risk of bleeding in some dogs. Subcutaneous enoxaparin, an LMWH, has been advocated in dogs at a rate of 1 mg/kg every 12 hours based on extrapolation from the human literature or at a dose of 0.8 mg/kg administered every 6 hours based on a pharmacokinetic study in normal dogs [28]. The use of dalteparin, another LMWH, was recently evaluated in six clinically ill dogs, and it was found that therapeutic levels could be achieved 3 hours after the subcutaneous administration of 150 U/kg [120]. No randomized controlled studies have documented the clinical efficacy of these recommendations for resolving PTE in veterinary patients.

The pathophysiology of pulmonary embolism in heartworm disease is somewhat different than that of PTE secondary to other disease conditions. Pulmonary embolism after treatment for heartworm infestation involves local inflammatory processes and losses in vascular endothelial integrity that are more comparable to the types of arteriosclerotic conditions in people for which aspirin therapy has been shown to be effective [38]. Evidence regarding the use of aspirin in dogs with heartworm disease, however, is contradictory and unclear. A 1981 study [121] evaluating the use of aspirin in canine pulmonary arteries damaged by short-term (4 days) or long-term (33 days) *Dirofilaria* infection concluded that aspirin was not effective in reducing platelet adhesion in the short term but did have beneficial long-term effects demonstrated by significant reductions in platelet adhesion after 30 days [121]. Another study in 1983 [122] compared aspirin and prednisone in therapy of pulmonary embolism in heartworm-affected dogs treated with thiacetarsamide and found that aspirin significantly reduced occlusion of the caudal pulmonary vasculature. A 1984 study evaluated aspirin and prednisone in postadulticide heartworm infection [123] and similarly found that that aspirin therapy led to improved pulmonary blood flow dynamics. In 1985, a study evaluated the effect of aspirin on year-long heartworm infections and concluded that aspirin had a protective effect against ongoing endothelial damage and dramatically reduced arteriosclerosis [124]. A 1991 study concluded that pulmonary vascular lesions in heartworm-infected dogs treated with aspirin or an aspirin-dipyridamole combination were not significantly different than those of control dogs, however [125]. Furthermore, a 1993 study evaluated the effects of prostaglandin inhibition on heartworm-related pulmonary vascular disease and concluded that prostaglandin inhibitors may be contraindicated [126]. In response to these more recent studies, the American Heartworm Society currently recommends that aspirin not be used in the treatment of heartworm-infected dogs [127].

With so little evidence regarding therapy for venous thrombosis and PTE in dogs and cats, many of our therapeutic decisions must be based on the clinical impressions of experts in the field, on pathophysiologic rationale, and on evidence extrapolated from human medicine. With this in mind, some therapeutic recommendations can be made for therapy in dogs and cats.

Recommendations for Maintenance Therapy for Pulmonary Thromboembolism in Small Animals

- For the therapy of venous thrombosis with or without PTE in dogs, warfarin may be considered at a dose of 0.22 mg/kg administered every 12 hours initially and then adjusted to achieve a PT prolongation of 1.25 to 1.5 times the pretreatment value.

- For the therapy of venous thrombosis with or without PTE in cats, warfarin may be considered at a dose of 0.5 mg/cat administered once daily initially and then adjusted to achieve a PT prolongation of 1.25 to 1.5 times the pretreatment value.
- Close monitoring of PT to ensure anticoagulant effect, to guard against bleeding, and to ensure owner and patient compliance is necessary with warfarin therapy.
- UFH should be administered concurrently with warfarin for the first 5 to 7 days of therapy, or at least until monitoring has documented adequate prolongation of PT. The recommended UFH dose in dogs is 200 to 500 U/kg administered subcutaneously every 8 hours initially and then adjusted to reach a target aPTT of 1.5 to 2 times the treatment values or anti-factor Xa activity between 0.35 and 0.70 U/mL.
- Enoxaparin or dalteparin may be considered as an alternative to warfarin therapy in dogs. The recommended dose for enoxaparin is 0.8 mg/kg administered subcutaneously every 6 hours. A reduced enoxaparin dose of 1 mg/kg administered every 12 hours may be considered to lessen expense and facilitate at-home administration, although anticoagulant efficacy at this dose has not been established in dogs. The suggested dose for dalteparin is 150 U/kg given subcutaneously every 12 hours. LMWH doses may be titrated by means of measurement of anti-Xa activity. No studies have evaluated the efficacy of LMWH in the resolution of naturally occurring PTE in dog or cats. Cost can be a significant issue with the LMWHs. Because a 300-mg vial of enoxaparin costs approximately $230 and a 10,000-U syringe of dalteparin costs approximately $60, treatment of a 20-kg dog at standard doses would cost approximately $12 or $20 a dose ($48 or $40 per day), respectively.
- For the treatment of PTE secondary to the treatment of heartworm disease in dogs, aspirin is not generally recommended.
- Additional recommendations for the management of existing venous thromboembolism and PTE in cats are similar to those for ATE.

PROPHYLACTIC THERAPY
Prophylactic Therapy in People
In human medicine, the list of risk factors for the development of venous thromboembolism is long (Box 1), and specific recommendations for prophylaxis are made for individual patients according to existing risk factors and concurrent disease. These recommendations apply to surgical, trauma, medical, and critical care patients as well as to patients with cancer and are further categorized according to individual types of disease or conditions.

General soft tissue surgery
The guidelines and recommendations for thromboprophylaxis in human surgical patients are extensive and beyond the scope of this review. Nevertheless, it is interesting to discuss some of these recommendations when they involve surgical procedures and conditions that are also commonly encountered in our veterinary patients. Surgical patients are considered to be at low risk for thromboembolism if they are undergoing a minor procedure and are young (<40

Box 1: Risk factors for thromboembolic complications in people

Surgery (risk varies with type and location of surgery)

Trauma (major or lower extremity)

Immobility, paresis

Cancer therapy (hormonal, chemotherapy, or radiation therapy)

Central venous catheterization

Acute medical illness

Heart or respiratory failure

Atrial fibrillation

Inflammatory bowel disease

Nephrotic syndrome

Myeloproliferative disorders

Paroxysmal nocturnal hemoglobinuria

Estrogen-containing oral contraceptive or hormone replacement therapy

Selective estrogen receptor modulators

Previous venous thrombosis

Pregnancy and postpartum period

Increased age

Obesity

Smoking

Varicose veins

Inherited or acquired thrombophilia

years of age) with no additional risk factors [53]. In these patients, no thrombo-prophylaxis is recommended. If the procedure is major, the patient is middle aged (between 40 and 60 years of age), or there is an additional predisposing factor for thromboembolism, the risk level is considered to be moderate and thromboprophylaxis in the form of low-dose UFH at 5000 U twice daily or LMWH at 3400 U or less once daily is recommended [53]. If the patient is undergoing a minor procedure and is older than 60 years of age or has an additional predisposing factor or if the patient is younger than 40 years of age but undergoing a major procedure or has an additional predisposing factor, the risk of thrombus formation is higher and thromboprophylaxis is recommended with UFH at 5000 U three times daily or LMWH at greater than 3400 U daily. In patients who have undergone major cancer surgery, long-term at-home therapy with LMWH is recommended. Thromboprophylaxis is recommended for all major urologic and gynecologic surgery and in the case of all patients undergoing laparoscopic surgery who have at least one other risk factor for thrombosis [53].

Orthopedic surgery
Major orthopedic surgery places patients at much greater risk for venous thrombosis than does other surgery, and routine thromboprophylaxis is recommended. Most symptomatic thrombi occur after discharge from the hospital, and the risk of thrombus formation remains elevated for as long as 2 months after surgery [128,129]. In spite of prophylactic therapy, thrombosis is the leading reason for hospital readmission after total hip replacement procedures [130]. Postsurgical asymptomatic deep vein thrombosis is common and is thought to affect at least 50% of human patients undergoing orthopedic surgery. Fortunately, most of these thrombi resolve spontaneously [131,132], although additional risk factors, such as persistent vascular injury, immobility [133], alterations in hemostasis [134,135], or a combination of these risk factors, may lead to propagation of the existing thrombus to the point that it becomes clinically significant and may lead to PTE.

For patients undergoing elective hip arthroplasty, thromboprophylaxis is recommended with LMWH started 12 hours before surgery or 12 to 24 hours after surgery or with warfarin started before or the evening after surgery. Similar thromboprophylaxis is recommended for elective knee arthroplasty and hip fracture surgery. Thromboprophylaxis is not routinely recommended for less major procedures, such as knee arthroscopy, unless the patient has other risk factors or the procedure was complicated and prolonged; in such cases, LMWH is advised [53].

Trauma, spinal cord injury, and burns
Thromboprophylaxis is recommended, whenever possible, in all major trauma patients with at least one risk factor for venous thrombosis. In the absence of major contraindications, LMWH should be started on admission to the hospital. Thromboprophylaxis should be continued until the patient is discharged from the hospital or longer in the case of people with significant impairment of mobility [53]. LMWH or UFH is recommended in all patients with acute spinal cord injury once primary hemostasis is found to be intact, and thromboprophylaxis with LMWH or warfarin should be continued during rehabilitation [53]. Low-dose UFH or LMWH is also suggested in all burn patients with one or more additional risk factors, including advanced age, morbid obesity, extensive lower extremity burns, concomitant lower extremity trauma, a femoral venous catheter, or prolonged immobility [53].

Medical conditions
Up to 70% of symptomatic thromboembolic events in people [136,137] and up to 80% of cases of fatal PTE occur in nonsurgical patients [138]. Hospitalization for any acute medical illness is associated with an eightfold higher relative risk for venous thrombosis [139]. Important risk factors for thrombosis in medical patients include advanced heart failure [140], chronic obstructive pulmonary disease exacerbations, sepsis, cancer, stroke with lower extremity weakness, a history of venous thrombosis, advanced age, and bed rest. Thromboprophylaxis is recommended in acutely ill patients admitted to the hospital with

congestive heart failure or severe respiratory disease and in patients who are confined to bed and have additional risk factors, such as active cancer, sepsis, acute neurologic disease, inflammatory bowel disease, or a history of thrombosis. UFH or LMWH is the therapy of choice [53].

Patients with cancer

There is a sixfold increase in the risk for venous thrombosis in patients with cancer compared with patients without cancer [139], and cancer underlies nearly 20% of all thromboses occurring outside the hospital [141]. There are few data, however, that help to predict which cancers carry the greatest risk for thrombosis. Known high-risk cancers include malignant brain tumors and ovarian, pancreatic, colonic, gastric, pulmonary, prostatic, and renal adenocarcinomas [142–144]. Patients with cancer undergoing surgery have nearly three times a greater risk for thrombosis than patients without cancer undergoing similar procedures [145]. Chemotherapy also increases the risk of thrombosis. In one study, patients receiving cytotoxic or immunosuppressive drugs had a 6.5-fold greater risk of thrombosis compared with patients without cancer [139]. Only one study [146] has evaluated the use of thromboprophylaxis in patients with cancer receiving chemotherapy, and it concluded that warfarin significantly decreased the incidence of venous thromboses, with no additional risk of bleeding in women with metastatic breast cancer. According to a recent review [53], however, there is not enough evidence available to make clear recommendations regarding thromboprophylaxis in most human patients with cancer.

Critical care patients

Two reviews have recently evaluated venous thromboses in populations of critical care patients [147,148] and have identified numerous risk factors that may be acquired during hospitalization, including immobilization, surgical procedures, central venous catheters, mechanical ventilation, renal dialysis, sedation, vasopressin administration, sepsis, heart failure, and depletion of anticoagulant factors. The reported incidence of deep vein thromboses in critical care human patients ranges from less than 10% to nearly 100%. Few studies have evaluated the use of thromboprophylaxis specifically in patients in the intensive care unit (ICU); however, one study evaluated the concurrent use of LMWH and vasopressor drugs and found that anti-factor Xa levels were significantly lower in patients who had been given vasopressors [149], presumably because of reduced absorption of the subcutaneous LMWH. Most patients in the ICU are considered to be at risk for developing venous thrombosis, and thromboprophylaxis is therefore indicated in most critical care patients. On admission to the ICU, it is recommended that patients be assessed for the risk of thrombosis and, accordingly, that most patients be started on anticoagulant therapy. Patients at moderate risk for thrombosis (medical or postoperative general surgery patients) should be started on low-dose UFH or LMWH, whereas those at higher risk (major trauma or orthopedic surgery) should be started on LMWH therapy [53].

Prophylactic Therapy in Small Animals

Evidence specific to the prevention of thromboembolic disease in at-risk patients is sparse in the veterinary literature. In recent years, more attention has been given to thromboembolic events as an important complication of several veterinary disease conditions; however, we must rely on the human literature and on pathophysiologic rationale for much of our information about the cause, pathophysiology, and therapy of thromboembolic disease. Unfortunately, however, those disease conditions associated with a high risk of thrombus formation in veterinary patients differ markedly from conditions associated with increased thrombotic risk in people in some instances. Little information is available on thromboprophylaxis for at-risk veterinary patients, and treatment has typically been reserved for patients with documented thrombosis or embolism.

Surgery

As is the case with human medicine, venous thrombosis or PTE that occurs as a result of surgery is often clinically silent, and little attention has been paid to thromboprophylactic therapy in veterinary surgical patients. Some of our surgical patients, however, may be at significant risk for clinical thromboembolism, and, as with human patients, risk factors may be cumulative. Rates of postsurgical thromboembolic events in small animals can certainly occur with a frequency that would warrant anticoagulant therapy in people. A 2003 study in dogs, for example, revealed that as many as 82% of animals undergoing total hip replacement surgery have evidence of pulmonary embolism after surgery [150]. Perioperative heparinization with UFH has recently been recommended for dogs undergoing adrenalectomy [151]. Anticoagulant therapy with the LMWH enoxaparin has also been recommended during the perioperative period in dogs undergoing renal transplantation [152].

Medical and critical care patients and patients with cancer

For most nonsurgical diseases in dogs and cats, the risk of thrombotic disease has not been typically been considered high enough to warrant routine thromboprophylaxis. There are several conditions [153–161], however, in which the risk of thrombotic complications is high enough to warrant consideration of preventative therapy. These conditions include protein-losing nephropathy, in which an incidence of thromboembolism as high as 25% has been reported in dogs [162]; immune-mediated hemolytic anemia (IMHA), which is associated with a PTE rate of 80% at necropsy [163]; and hypertrophic cardiomyopathy in cats, with an incidence of ATE as high as 33% to 50% [109,164].

Thromboprophylactic therapy is currently routinely recommended in cases of canine protein-losing nephropathy and nephrotic syndrome [165]. The prothrombotic state associated with nephrotic syndrome is likely to attributable to several abnormalities in the hemostatic system. Antithrombin deficiency secondary to renal losses is often implicated as the key causative factor but is unlikely to be the sole factor contributing to thrombosis with nephrotic syndrome [166]. Platelets may also play a role in the prothrombotic state seen with nephrotic syndrome; protein-losing nephropathies are often associated with thrombocytosis and increased platelet adhesion and aggregation [167]. Low-dose aspirin therapy (0.5–5 mg/kg once to twice daily) has therefore been advocated in the therapy of glomerulonephritis and nephrotic syndrome in dogs [165]. Protein-losing enteropathies have also been associated with losses in antithrombin and with hypercoagulable states [168,169] potentially leading to thromboembolism, but no specific treatment recommendations have been made.

Hyperadrenocorticism has also been clearly associated with an increased risk of thromboembolic complications, particularly PTE [170]. The incidence of PTE in dogs with hyperadrenocorticism is probably not high enough to warrant routine thromboprophylaxis. Prophylactic therapy is, however, recommended in the face of additional risk factors, such as major surgery.

IMHA in dogs is complicated by a hypercoagulable state in as many as 50% of the dogs at the time of diagnosis [163,171]. PTE, in particular, is well recognized to be a major cause of mortality in dogs with IMHA [163,172,173]. To date, however, only one clinical trial has evaluated the use of thromboprophylactic drug therapy in dogs with IMHA. This 2005 retrospective study compared the use of ultralow-dose aspirin (0.5 mg/kg/d), UFH, or a combination of the two and found that dogs that received aspirin had significantly better survival rates than dogs that did not [174].

As many as 50% of cats with hypertrophic cardiomyopathy go on to develop ATE. Aspirin therapy has been recommended as thromboprophylactic therapy in feline ATE at a dose of 81 mg per cat administered orally every 48 to 72 hours [97,98]. A more recent study, however, has suggested that a lower dose of 5 mg per cat administered every 72 hours is just as effective in preventing recurrence of ATE and has fewer side effects than the higher dose aspirin [99]. This low-dose aspirin protocol could reasonably be used as prophylaxis in cats at risk for a first ATE episode. Warfarin has also been advocated for use in preventing ATE in at-risk cats before a first embolic episode at doses similar to those suggested for the treatment of existing ATE. No studies are available that clearly document the efficacy of any prophylactic therapy in preventing ATE in cats, however.

Disseminated intravascular coagulation (DIC), a state of increased hypercoagulability and excessive small thrombus formation that leads to eventual consumptive of platelets and clotting factors, should also be considered in a discussion of thromboembolic therapy. DIC can occur secondary to a diverse range of different disease states. Heparinization has been advocated for human patients with DIC, although the efficacy of heparin therapy is uncertain, because there have been few controlled clinical studies [175]. Heparin has also been advocated in dogs with DIC, using low-dose (75 U/kg every 8 hours) and high-dose (200 U/kg every 6 hours) protocols, but no controlled studies have evaluated the efficacy of either protocol in improving clinical outcome. High-dose heparin protocols have been evaluated in experimental and naturally occurring DIC in dogs, with some favorable results with respect to improvement in laboratory abnormalities but with no reduction in overall mortality [175,176]. Antithrombin deficiency has been implicated as a cause of some of the coagulation abnormalities seen with DIC, and the use of plasma as a source of antithrombin has therefore also been advocated in human [177] and veterinary patients with DIC [175]. One recent study evaluated the use of LMWH in dogs with experimentally induced DIC and concluded that LMWH effectively interrupted consumptive processes if administered at a dose sufficient to achieve anti-factor Xa levels between approximately 0.6 and 0.9 U/mL [178]. Although there are considerable pathophysiologic data demonstrating a hypercoagulable state in veterinary patients with cancer [179], there have been no studies evaluating the use of thromboprophylaxis in small animals with cancer.

Although there are few studies evaluating thromboprophylaxis in the veterinary medical literature, some recommendations can be made based on the information available from the human literature, from pathophysiologic rationale, and on recommendations based on the clinical experience of experts in the field.

Recommendations for Prophylactic Therapy in Small Animals

- Perioperative or postoperative thromboprophylaxis should be considered in patients undergoing major operations that are associated with a high rate of thrombosis in people (eg, major hip surgery) or in patients that have additional risk factors for thromboembolic disease, such as cancer.
- Specifically, hyperadrenocorticoid dogs undergoing adrenalectomy should be treated with heparinized plasma at a rate of 35 U/kg at anesthetic induction, followed by two additional doses of subcutaneous heparin at 35 U/kg on the day of surgery (8 hours apart), followed by 25 U/kg every 8 hours the next day and then tapered over the next 4 days.
- Aspirin at a dose of 0.5 to 5 mg/kg administered once or twice daily should be considered in the treatment of dogs with protein-losing nephropathy and nephrotic syndrome.
- Aspirin at a dose of 0.5 mg/kg/d is recommended for dogs with IMHA.
- Aspirin at a dose of 5 mg per cat can be considered for the prevention of ATE in at-risk cats, although no studies have documented the efficacy of this approach.
- Warfarin therapy has been suggested for preventing ATE in at-risk cats, although there are no studies confirming the efficacy of this or any other anticoagulant therapy in preventing a first occurrence of ATE.
- Thromboprophylactic therapy should be considered in patients with protein-losing enteropathy or hyperadrenocorticism if further risk factors for thromboembolic disease exist.

SUMMARY OF RECOMMENDATIONS: SPECIFIC DISEASE CONDITIONS

Feline Aortic Thromboembolism
- Thrombolytic therapy should not be used.
- Dietary supplementation with n-3 fatty acids is not recommended.
- Aspirin is recommended at a dose of 5 mg/kg administered every 72 hours.

- Subcutaneous UFH at a dose of 250 to 300 U/kg administered every 8 hours is recommended during initial therapy.
- LMWH may also be considered, especially for long-term management, although there is no evidence supporting the benefit of LMWH over aspirin alone or aspirin and LMWH combined.
- Aspirin at a dose of 5 mg per cat is recommended for the prevention of ATE in at-risk cats.
- Clopidogrel is not recommended as adjunct therapy for clot lysis but may potentially prove to be a reasonable alternative to aspirin for long-term control.

Canine Immune-Mediated Hemolytic Anemia

- Aspirin therapy at a dose of 0.5 mg/kg/d is recommended.
- Although many heparinization protocols have been suggested for dogs with IMHA, including constant rate infusions with UFH, subcutaneous heparin at various doses, and LMWH (eg, enoxaparin, dalteparin), there is, to date, no evidence that such therapy reduces the incidence of PTE. Given the high incidence of life-threatening PTE in patients with IMHA, there is clearly a need to identify and aggressively explore anticoagulant strategies that reduce the incidence of thrombotic complications.

Protein-Losing Nephropathy in Dogs

- Aspirin at a dose of 0.5 to 5 mg/kg administered once or twice daily should be considered.

Protein-Losing Enteropathy

- Thromboprophylactic therapy should be considered in patients with other risk factors for thromboembolic disease.

Hyperadrenocorticism

- Thromboprophylactic therapy should be considered in patients with other risk factors for thromboembolic disease.

Surgical Patients

- Perioperative thromboprophylactic therapy should be considered in patients undergoing major surgery, especially in those that have additional risk factors for thrombosis.
- Dogs undergoing adrenalectomy for hyperadrenocorticism should be treated with perioperative heparinized plasma and subcutaneous UFH.

References

[1] Hirsh J, Guyatt G, Albers GW, et al. The Seventh ACCP Conference on Antithrombotic and Thrombolytic Therapy: evidence based guidelines. Chest 2004;126:172–3.
[2] Schünemann HJ, Munger H, Brower S, et al. Methodology for guideline development for the Seventh American College of Chest Physicians Conference of Antithrombotic and Thrombolytic Therapy. Chest 2004;126:174–8.
[3] Guyatt G, Schünemann HJ, Cook D, et al. Applying the grades of recommendation for antithrombotic and thrombolytic therapy: the Seventh ACCP Conference of Antithrombotic and Thrombolytic Therapy. Chest 2004;126:179–87.
[4] Marjerus PW, Broze GJ Jr, Miletich JP, et al. Anticoagulant, thrombolytic, and antiplatelet drugs. In: Hardman JG, Limbird LE, Molinoff PB, et al, editors. Goodman and Gilman's the pharmacologic basis of therapeutics. 9th edition. New York: McGraw-Hill; 1996. p. 1341–59.

[5] Roth GJ, Majerus PW. The mechanism of the effect of aspirin on human platelets: I. Acetylation of a particulate fraction protein. J Clin Invest 1975;56:624–32.

[6] Majerus PW. Arachidonate metabolism in vascular disorders. J Clin Invest 1983;72: 1521–5.

[7] Clarke RJ, Mayo G, Price P, et al. Suppression of thromboxane A$_2$ but not systemic prostacyclin by controlled-release aspirin. N Engl J Med 1991;325:1137–41.

[8] McAdam BF, Catella-Lawson F, Mardini IA, et al. Systemic biosynthesis of prostacyclin by cyclooxygenase (COX)-2: the human pharmacology of a selective inhibitor of COX-2. Proc Natl Acad Sci U S A 1999;96:272–7.

[9] Cipollone F, Patrignani P, Greco A, et al. Differential suppression of thromboxane biosynthesis by indobufen and aspirin in patients with unstable angina. Circulation 1997;96: 1109–16.

[10] Preston FE, Whipps S, Jackson CA, et al. Inhibition of prostacyclin and platelet thromboxane A$_2$ after low-dose aspirin. N Engl J Med 1981;304:76–9.

[11] Patrignani P, Filabozzi P, Patrono C. Selective cumulative inhibition of platelet thromboxane production by low-dose aspirin in healthy subjects. J Clin Invest 1982;69:1366–72.

[12] Patrono C. Aspirin as an antiplatelet drug. N Engl J Med 1994;330:1287–94.

[13] Quinn MJ, Fitzgerald DJ. Ticlopidine and clopidogrel. Circulation 1999;100:1667–72.

[14] Hogan DF, Andrews DA, Green HW, et al. Antiplatelet effects and pharmacodynamics of clopidogrel in cats. J Am Vet Med Assoc 2004;225(9):1406–11.

[15] Hirsch J, Raschke R. Heparin and low molecular weight heparins: the Seventh ACCP Conference on Antithrombotic and Thrombolytic Therapy. Chest 2004;126:188S–203S.

[16] Johnson EA, Mulloy B. The molecular weight range of commercial heparin preparations. Carbohydr Res 1976;51:119–27.

[17] Lam LH, Silbert JE, Rosenberg RD. The separation of active and inactive forms of heparin. Biochem Biophys Res Commun 1976;69:570–7.

[18] Casu B, Oreste P, Torri G, et al. The structure of heparin oligosaccharide fragments with high anti-(factor Xa) activity containing the minimal antithrombin III-binding sequence. Biochem J 1981;97:599–609.

[19] Ofosu FA, Sie P, Modi GJ, et al. The inhibition of thrombin-dependent feedback reactions is critical to the expression of anticoagulant effects of heparin. Biochem J 1987;243: 579–88.

[20] Ofosu FA, Hirsh J, Esmon CT, et al. Unfractionated heparin inhibits thrombin-catalyzed amplification reactions of coagulation more efficiently than those catalyzed by factor Xa. Biochem J 1989;257:143–50.

[21] Beguin S, Lindhout T, Hemker HC. The mode of action of heparin in plasma. Thromb Haemost 1988;60:457–62.

[22] Mischke RH, Schuttert C, Grebe SI. Anticoagulant effects of repeated subcutaneous injections of high doses of unfractionated heparin in healthy dogs. Am J Vet Res 2001;62(12): 1887–91.

[23] Harenberg J. Pharmacology of low molecular weight heparins. Semin Thromb Hemost 1990;16:12–8.

[24] Hirsh J, Levine MN. Low molecular weight heparin. Blood 1992;79:1–17.

[25] Handeland GF, Abidgaard GF, Holm U, et al. Dose adjusted heparin treatment of deep venous thrombosis: a comparison of unfractionated and low molecular weight heparin. Eur J Clin Pharmacol 1990;39:107–12.

[26] Abbate R, Gori AM, Farsi A, et al. Monitoring of low-molecular-weight heparins. Am J Cardiol 1998;82:33L–6L.

[27] Levine MN, Planes A, Hirsh J, et al. The relationship between antifactor Xa level and clinical outcome in patients receiving enoxaparin low molecular weight heparin to prevent deep vein thrombosis after hip replacement. Thromb Haemost 1989;62:940–4.

[28] Lunsford K, Mackin A, Langston VC, et al. Pharmacokinetics of the biological effects of subcutaneously administered enoxaparin, a low molecular weight heparin, in dogs [abstract].

Presented at the Proceedings of the American College of Veterinary Internal Medicine. 2005.

[29] Mischke R, Grebe S, Jacobs C, et al. Amidolytic heparin activity and values for several hemostatic variables after repeated subcutaneous administration of high doses of a low molecular weight heparin in healthy dogs. Am J Vet Res 2001;62(4):595–8.

[30] Ansell J, Hirsch J, Poller L, et al. The pharmacology and management of vitamin K antagonists: the seventh ACCP conference on antithrombotic and thrombolytic therapy. Chest 2004;126:204S–33S.

[31] Fasco MJ, Hildebrandt EF, Suttie JW. Evidence that warfarin anticoagulant action involves two distinct reductase activities. J Biol Chem 1982;257:11210–2.

[32] Nelsestuen GL, Zytkovicz TH, Howard JB. The mode of action of vitamin K: identification of γ-carboxyglutamic acid as a component of prothrombin. J Biol Chem 1974;249:6347–50.

[33] Hirsh J, Dalen JE, Anderson DR, et al. Oral anticoagulants: mechanism of action, clinical effectiveness, and optimal therapeutic range. Chest 2001;119(Suppl):8S–21S.

[34] Nelsestuen GL. Role of gamma-carboxyglutamic acid: an unusual transition required for calcium-dependent binding of prothrombin to phospholipid. J Biol Chem 1976;251: 5648–56.

[35] Borowski M, Furie BC, Bauminger S, et al. Prothrombin requires two sequential metal-dependent conformational transitions to bind phospholipid. J Biol Chem 1986;261: 14969–75.

[36] Kelly JG, O'Malley K. Clinical pharmacokinetics of oral anticoagulants. Clin Pharmacokinet 1979;4:1–15.

[37] Kirkwood TBL. Calibration of reference thromboplastins and standardisation of the prothrombin time ratio. Thromb Haemost 1983;49:238–44.

[38] Clagett GP, Sobel M, Jackson MR, et al. Antithrombotic therapy in peripheral arterial occlusive disease: the Seventh ACCP Conference on Antithrombotic and Thrombolytic Therapy. Chest 2004;126:609S–26S.

[39] Davidian MM, Powell A, Benenati J, et al. Initial results of reteplase in the treatment of acute lower extremity arterial occlusions. J Vasc Interv Radiol 2000;11:289–94.

[40] Ouriel K, Katzen B, Mewissen M, et al. Reteplase in the treatment of peripheral arterial and venous occlusions: a pilot study. J Vasc Interv Radiol 2000;11:849–54.

[41] Berridge DC, Gregson RHS, Hopkinson BR, et al. Randomized trial of intra-arterial recombinant tissue plasminogen activator, intravenous recombinant tissue plasminogen activator and intra-arterial streptokinase in peripheral arterial thrombolysis. Br J Surg 1991;78:988–95.

[42] Meyerovitz MF, Goldhaber SZ, Reagan K, et al. Recombinant tissue-type plasminogen activator versus urokinase in peripheral arterial and graft occlusions: a randomized trial. Radiology 1990;175:75–8.

[43] The STILE Investigators. Results of a prospective randomized trial evaluating surgery versus thrombolysis for ischemia of the lower extremity: the STILE trial. Ann Surg 1994;220: 251–68.

[44] Schweizer J, Altmann E, Florek HJ, et al. Comparison of tissue plasminogen activator and urokinase in the local infiltration thrombolysis of peripheral arterial occlusions. Eur J Radiol 1996;23:64–73.

[45] Palfrayman SJ, Booth A, Michaels JA. A systematic review of intra-arterial thrombolytic therapy for lower-limb ischaemia. Eur J Vasc Endovasc Surg 2000;19:143–57.

[46] Berridge DC, Kessel D, Robertson I. Surgery versus thrombolysis for acute limb ischaemia: initial management. Cochrane Database Syst Rev 2002;1:CD002784.

[47] Nilsson L, Albrechtsson U, Jonung T, et al. Surgical treatment versus thrombolysis in acute arterial occlusion: a randomized controlled study. Eur J Vasc Surg 1992;6:189–93.

[48] Ouriel K, Shortell CK, De Weese JA, et al. A comparison of thrombolytic therapy with operative vascularization in the initial treatment of acute peripheral arterial ischemia. J Vasc Surg 1994;19:1021–30.

[49] Weaver FA, Comerota AJ, Youngblood M, et al. Surgical revascularization versus thrombolysis for nonembolic lower extremity native artery occlusions: results of a prospective randomized trial. J Vasc Surg 1996;24:513–21.

[50] Comerota AJ, Weaver FA, Hosking JD, et al. Results of prospective, randomized trial of surgery versus thrombolysis for occluded lower extremity bypass grafts. Am J Surg 1996;172: 105–12.

[51] Ouriel K, Veith FJ, Sasahara AA. Thrombolysis or peripheral arterial surgery: phase I results. J Vasc Surg 1996;23:64–75.

[52] Ouriel K, Veith FJ, Sasahara AA. A comparison of recombinant urokinase with vascular surgery as initial treatment for acute arterial occlusion of the legs. N Engl J Med 1998;338: 1105–11.

[53] Geerts WH, Pineo GF, Heit JA, et al. Prevention of venous thromboembolism: the Seventh ACCP Conference on Antithrombotic and Thrombolytic Therapy. Chest 2004;126: 338S–400S.

[54] Goldhaber SZ, Meyerovitz MF, Green D, et al. Randomized controlled trial of tissue plasminogen activator in proximal deep venous thrombosis. Am J Med 1990;88:235–40.

[55] Lensing AW, Hirsh J. Rationale and results of thrombolytic therapy for deep vein thrombosis. In: Bernstein EF, editor. Vascular diagnosis. 4th edition. St. Louis (MO): Mosby; 1994. p. 875–9.

[56] Goldhaber SZ, Kessler CM, Heit J, et al. Randomised controlled trial of recombinant tissue plasminogen activator versus urokinase in the treatment of acute pulmonary embolism. Lancet 1988;2:293–8.

[57] Bell WR, Simon TL, Stengle JM, et al. Urokinase pulmonary embolism trial: phase 1 results; a cooperative study. JAMA 1970;214:2163–72.

[58] Urokinase-streptokinase embolism trial: phase 2 results; a cooperative study. JAMA 1974;229:1606–13.

[59] Moore KE, Morris N, Dhupa N, et al. Retrospective study of streptokinase administration in 46 cats with arterial thromboembolism. Journal of Veterinary Emergency and Critical Care 2000;10(4):245–57.

[60] Anderson DR, Levine MN. Thrombolytic therapy for the treatment of acute pulmonary embolism. Can Med Assoc J 1992;146:1317–24.

[61] The Columbus Investigators. Low-molecular-weight heparin in the treatment of patients with venous thromboembolism. N Engl J Med 1997;337:657–62.

[62] Douketis JD, Kearon C, Bates S, et al. Risk of fatal pulmonary embolism in patients with treated venous thromboembolism. JAMA 1998;279:458–62.

[63] Hull RD, Raskob GE, Brant RF, et al. Low-molecular-weight heparin vs heparin in the treatment of patients with pulmonary embolism: American-Canadian Thrombosis Study Group. Arch Intern Med 2000;160:229–36.

[64] Simonneau G, Sors H, Charbonnier B, et al. A comparison of low-molecular-weight heparin with unfractionated heparin for acute pulmonary embolism. N Engl J Med 1997;337: 663–9.

[65] Carson JL, Kelley MA, Duff A, et al. The clinical course of pulmonary embolism. N Engl J Med 1992;326:1240–5.

[66] Sharma GV, Burleson VA, Sasahara AA. Effect of thrombolytic therapy on pulmonary-capillary blood volume in patients with pulmonary embolism. N Engl J Med 1980;303: 842–5.

[67] Thompson MF, Scott-Moncrieff JC, Hogan DF. Thrombolytic therapy in dogs and cats. Journal of Veterinary Emergency and Critical Care 2001;11(2):111–21.

[68] Killingsworth CR, Eyster GE, Adams T, et al. Streptokinase treatment of cats with experimentally induced aortic thrombosis. Am J Vet Res 1986;47(6):1351–9.

[69] Ramsey CC, Riepe RD, Macintire DK, et al. Streptokinase: a practical clot buster? Proceedings, Fifth International Veterinary Emergency and Critical Care Symposium. San Antonio, TX 1996; 225–228.

[70] Pion PD. Feline aortic thromboemboli and the potential utility of thrombolytic therapy with tissue plasminogen activator. Vet Clin North Am Small Anim Pract 1988;18(1):79–86.

[71] Fox PR. Feline thromboembolism associated with cardiomyopathy. Proceedings of the Fifth Annual Veterinary Medical Forum ACVIM 1987; 714–718.

[72] Ramsey CC, Burney DP, Macintire DK, et al. Use of streptokinase in four dogs with thrombosis. J Am Vet Med Assoc 1996;209(4):780–5.

[73] Tater KC, Drellich S, Beck K. Management of femoral artery thrombosis in an immature dog. Journal of Veterinary Emergency and Critical Care 2005;15(1):52–9.

[74] Clare AC, Kraje BJ. Use of tissue recombinant tissue-plasminogen activator for aortic thrombolysis in a hypoproteinemic dog. J Am Vet Med Assoc 1998;212(4):439–43.

[75] Bliss SP, Bliss SK, Harvey HJ. Use of recombinant tissue-plasminogen activator in a dog with chylothorax secondary to catheter-associated thrombosis of the cranial vena cava. J Am Anim Hosp Assoc 2002;38(5):431–5.

[76] Hull R, Pineo G, Mah A, et al. A randomized trial evaluating longterm low-molecular-weight heparin therapy for three months versus intravenous heparin followed by warfarin sodium [abstract]. Blood 2002;100:148a.

[77] Büller HR, Agnelli G, Hull RD, et al. Antithrombotic therapy for venous thromboembolic disease: the Seventh ACCP Conference on Antithrombotic and Thrombolytic Therapy. Chest 2004;126:410S–28S.

[78] Anand SS, Bates S, Ginsberg JS, et al. Recurrent venous thrombosis and heparin therapy: an evaluation of the importance of early activated partial thromboplastin times. Arch Intern Med 1999;159:2029–32.

[79] Levine MN, Raskob G, Landefeld S, et al. Hemorrhagic complications of anticoagulant treatment. Chest 2001;119(Suppl):108S–21S.

[80] Hommes DW, Bura A, Mazzolai L, et al. Subcutaneous heparin compared with continuous intravenous heparin administration in the initial treatment of deep vein thrombosis: a meta-analysis. Ann Intern Med 1992;116:279–84.

[81] Hull R, Delmore T, Carter C, et al. Adjusted subcutaneous heparin versus warfarin sodium in the long-term treatment of venous thrombosis. N Engl J Med 1982;306:189–94.

[82] Levine M, Gent M, Hirsh J, et al. A comparison of low-molecular-weight heparin administered primarily at home with unfractionated heparin administered in the hospital for proximal deep-vein thrombosis. N Engl J Med 1996;334:677–81.

[83] Koopman MM, Prandoni P, Piovella F, et al. Treatment of venous thrombosis with intravenous unfractionated heparin administered in the hospital as compared with subcutaneous low-molecular-weight heparin administered at home: the Tasman Study Group. N Engl J Med 1996;334:682–7.

[84] Merli G, Spiro TE, Olsson CG, et al. Subcutaneous enoxaparin once or twice daily compared with intravenous unfractionated heparin for treatment of venous thromboembolic disease. Ann Intern Med 2001;134:191–202.

[85] Charbonnier BA, Fiessinger JN, Banga JD, et al. Comparison of a once daily with a twice daily subcutaneous low molecular weight heparin regimen in the treatment of deep vein thrombosis. Thromb Haemost 1998;79:897–901.

[86] Hull R, Pineo GF, Mah A, et al. Safety and efficacy results for a study investigating the long-term out-of-hospital treatment of patients with proximal-vein thrombosis using subcutaneous low-molecular-weight heparin versus warfarin. Thromb Haemost 2001;1(Suppl 1):abstract OC1647.

[87] Lee AY, Levine MN, Baker RI, et al. Low-molecular-weight heparin versus a coumarin for the prevention of recurrent venous thromboembolism in patients with cancer. N Engl J Med 2003;349:146–53.

[88] Lagerstedt CI, Olsson CG, Fagher BO, et al. Need for long-term anticoagulant treatment in symptomatic calf-vein thrombosis. Lancet 1985;2:515–8.

[89] Hull R, Delmore T, Genton E, et al. Warfarin sodium versus low-dose heparin in the long-term treatment of venous thrombosis. N Engl J Med 1979;301:855–8.

[90] Ridker PM, Goldhaber SZ, Danielson E, et al. Long-term, low-intensity warfarin therapy for the prevention of recurrent venous thromboembolism. N Engl J Med 2003;348:1425–34.

[91] Kearon C, Ginsberg JS, Kovacs MJ, et al. Comparison of low-intensity warfarin therapy with conventional-intensity warfarin therapy for long-term prevention of recurrent venous thromboembolism. N Engl J Med 2003;349:631–9.

[92] Hull R, Hirsh J, Jay R, et al. Different intensities of oral anticoagulant therapy in the treatment of proximal-vein thrombosis. N Engl J Med 1982;307:1676–81.

[93] Crowther MA, Ginsberg JS, Julian J, et al. A comparison of two intensities of warfarin for the prevention of recurrent thrombosis in patients with the antiphospholipid antibody syndrome. N Engl J Med 2003;349:1133–8.

[94] Eichinger S, Minar E, Bialonczyk C, et al. D-dimer levels and risk of recurrent venous thromboembolism. J Am Med Assoc 2003;290:1071–4.

[95] Bright JM, Sullivan PS, Melton SL, et al. The effects of n-3 fatty acid supplementation on bleeding time, plasma fatty acid composition, and in vitro platelet aggregation in cats. J Vet Intern Med 1994;8(4):247–52.

[96] Boudreaux MK, Reinhart GA, Vaughn DM, et al. The effects of varying dietary n-6 to n-3 fatty acid ratios on platelet reactivity, coagulation screening assays, and antithrombin III activity in dogs. J Am Anim Hosp Assoc 1997;33(3):235–43.

[97] Flanders JA. Feline aortic thromboembolism. Compendium on Continuing Education for the Practicing Veterinarian 1986;8(7):473–83.

[98] Fox PR. Evidence for or against efficacy of beta-blockers and aspirin for management of feline cardiomyopathies. Vet Clin N Am Small Anim Pract 1991;21(5):1011–22.

[99] Smith SA, Tobias AH, Jacob KA, et al. Arterial thromboembolism in cats: acute crisis in 127 cases (1992–2001) and long-term management with low-dose aspirin in 24 cases. J Vet Intern Med 2003;17(1):73–83.

[100] Boswood A, Lamb CR, White RN. Aortic and iliac thrombosis in six dogs. J Small Anim Pract 2000;41(3):109–14.

[101] Fox PR, Petrie JP, Hohenhaus AE. Peripheral vascular disease. In: Ettinger SJ, Feldman EC, editors. Textbook of veterinary internal medicine. 6th edition. Philadelphia: WB Saunders; 2004. p. 1149–50.

[102] Harpster NK, Baty CJ. Warfarin therapy of the cat at risk of thromboembolism. In: Bonagura JD, editor. Kirk's current veterinary therapy XII. Philadelphia: WB Saunders; 1995. p. 868–73.

[103] Atkins CE. Therapy of feline heart disease. Presented at the 77th Annual Western Veterinary Conference. Las Vegas, NV, 2005.

[104] Smith SA, Kraft SL, Lewis DC, et al. Plasma pharmacokinetics of warfarin enantiomers in cats. J Vet Pharmacol Ther 2000;23(6):329–37.

[105] Smith SA, Kraft SL, Lewis DC, et al. Pharmacodynamics of warfarin in cats. J Vet Pharmacol Ther 2000;23(6):339–44.

[106] Smith SA, Tobias AH. Feline arterial thromboembolism: an update. Vet Clin North Am Small Anim Pract 2004;34(5):1245–71.

[107] DeFrancesco TC, Moore RR, Atkins CE, et al. Comparison of dalteparin and warfarin in the long-term management of feline arterial thromboembolism. Presented at the ACVIM annual meeting. Charlotte, NC, 2003.

[108] Smith CE, Rozanski EA, Freeman LM, et al. Use of low molecular weight heparin in cats: 57 cases (1999–2003). J Am Vet Med Assoc 2004;225(8):1237–41.

[109] Rush JE, Freeman LM, Fenollosa NK, et al. Population and survival characteristics of cats with hypertrophic cardiomyopathy: 260 cases (1990–1999). J Am Vet Med Assoc 2002;220:202–7.

[110] Laste NJ, Harpster NK. A retrospective study of 100 cases of feline distal aortic thromboembolism: 1977–1993. J Am Anim Hosp Assoc 1995;31:492–522.

[111] Pion PD, Kittleson MD. Therapy for feline aortic thromboembolism. In: Kirk RW, editor. Current veterinary therapy X. Philadelphia: WB Saunders; 1989. p. 295–302.

[112] Hogan DF, Ward MP. Effect of clopidogrel on tissue-plasminogen activator induced in vitro thrombolysis of feline whole blood thrombi. Am J Vet Res 2004;65(6): 715–9.

[113] Smith SA. Warfarin treatment in small animal patients [abstract]. Proceedings of the 16th Annual ACVIM Forum, American College of Veterinary Internal Medicine, San Diego, 1998. p. 440.

[114] Monnet E, Morgan MR. Effect of three loading doses of warfarin on the international normalized ratio for dogs. Am J Vet Res 2000;61(1):48–50.

[115] Rosanski E. Management of the hyper-coagulable patient, anticoagulant therapy. Tufts animal expo 2002. Presented at the Tufts Animal Expo. North Grafton, MA, 2002.

[116] Brooks M. Coagulopathies and thrombosis. In: Ettinger S, Feldman E, editors. Textbook of veterinary internal medicine. diseases of the dog and cat Vol. 2. Philadelphia: WB Saunders; 2000. p. 1829–41.

[117] Smith SA, Lewis DC, Kellerman DL. Adjustment of intermittent subcutaneous heparin therapy based on chromogenic heparin assay in 9 cats with thromboembolic disease [abstract]. J Vet Intern Med 1998;12:200.

[118] Kellerman DL, Lewis DC, Bruyette DS, et al. Determination and monitoring of a therapeutic heparin dosage in the dog [abstract]. J Vet Intern Med 1995;9:187.

[119] Brooks MB. Evaluation of a chromogenic assay to measure the factor Xa inhibitory activity of unfractionated heparin in canine plasma. Vet Clin Pathol 2004;33(4):208–14.

[120] Dunn M, Charland V, Thorneloe C. The use of a low molecular weight heparin in 6 dogs. Presented at the ACVIM annual meeting. Minneapolis, MN, June 2004.

[121] Schaub RG, Rawlings CA. Effects of long-term aspirin treatment on platelet adhesion to chronically damaged canine pulmonary arteries. Thromb Haemost 1981;46(4):680–3.

[122] Keith JC Jr, Rawlings CA, Schaub RG. Pulmonary thromboembolism during therapy of dirofilariasis with thiacetarsamide: modification with aspirin or prednisone. Am J Vet Res 1983;44(7):1278–83.

[123] Rawlings CA, Keith JC Jr, Losonsky JM, et al. An aspirin-prednisolone combination to modify postadulticide lung disease in heartworm-infected dogs. Am J Vet Res 1984;45(11):2371–5.

[124] Rawlings CA, Keith JC Jr, Schaub RG. Effect of acetylsalicylic acid on pulmonary arteriosclerosis induced by a one-year Dirofilaria immitis infection. Arteriosclerosis 1985;5(4): 355–65.

[125] Boudreaux MK, Dillon AR, Ravis WR, et al. Effects of treatment with aspirin or aspirin/dipyridamole combination in heartworm-negative, heartworm-infected, and embolized heartworm infected dogs. Am J Vet Res 1991;52(12):1992–9.

[126] Tarish JH, Atwell RB. The effect of prostaglandin inhibition on the development of pulmonary pathology associated with dead Dirofilaria immitis. Vet Parasitol 1993;49(2–4): 207–17.

[127] 2005 guidelines for the diagnosis, prevention and management of heartworm (Dirofilaria immitis) infection in dogs. American Heartworm Society Available at: http://www.heartwormsociety.org/. Accessed September 2006.

[128] Douketis JD, Eikelboom JW, Quinlan DJ, et al. Short-duration prophylaxis against venous thromboembolism after total hip or knee replacement: a meta-analysis of prospective studies investigating symptomatic outcomes. Arch Intern Med 2002;162:1465–71.

[129] White RH, Romano PS, Zhou H, et al. Incidence and time course of thromboembolic outcomes following total hip or knee arthroplasty. Arch Intern Med 1998;158:1525–31.

[130] Seagroatt V, Tan HS, Goldacre M. Elective total hip replacement: incidence, emergency readmission rate, and postoperative mortality. BMJ 1991;303:1431–5.

[131] Ginsberg JS, Gent M, Turkstra F, et al. Postthrombotic syndrome after hip or knee arthroplasty: a cross-sectional study. Arch Intern Med 2000;160:669–72.

[132] Kim YH, Oh SH, Kim JS. Incidence and natural history of deep-vein thrombosis after total hip arthroplasty. J Bone Joint Surg Br 2003;85:661–5.

[133] Buehler KO, D'Lima DD, Petersilge WJ, et al. Late deep venous thrombosis and delayed weight bearing after total hip arthroplasty. Clin Orthop 1999;361:123–30.

[134] Lindahl TL, Lundahl TH, Nilsson L, et al. APC-resistance is a risk factor for postoperative thromboembolism in elective replacement of the hip or knee: a prospective study. Thromb Haemost 1999;81:18–21.

[135] Westrich GH, Weksler BB, Glueck CJ, et al. Correlation of thrombophilia and hypofibrinolysis with pulmonary embolism following total hip arthroplasty: an analysis of genetic factors. J Bone Joint Surg Am 2002;84:2161–7.

[136] Bouthier J. The venous thrombotic risk in nonsurgical patients. Drugs 1996;52(Suppl): 16–29.

[137] Goldhaber SZ, Dunn K, MacDougall RC, et al. New onset of venous thromboembolism among hospitalized patients at Brigham and Women's Hospital is caused more often by prophylaxis failure than by withholding treatment. Chest 2000;118:1680–4.

[138] Alikhan R, Peters F, Wilmott R, et al. Epidemiology of fatal pulmonary embolism in nonsurgical patients [abstract]. Blood 2002;100:276a.

[139] Heit JA, Silverstein MD, Mohr DN, et al. Risk factors for deep vein thrombosis and pulmonary embolism: a population-based case-control study. Arch Intern Med 2000;160: 809–15.

[140] Howell MD, Geraci JM, Knowlton AA. Congestive heart failure and outpatient risk of venous thromboembolism: a retrospective, case-control study. J Clin Epidemiol 2001;54: 810–6.

[141] Heit JA, O'Fallon WM, Petterson TM, et al. Relative impact of risk factors for deep vein thrombosis and pulmonary embolism: a population-based study. Arch Intern Med 2002; 162:1245–8.

[142] Levitan N, Dowlati A, Remick SC, et al. Rates of initial and recurrent thromboembolic disease among patients with malignancy versus those without malignancy: risk analysis using Medicare claims data. Medicine 1999;78:285–91.

[143] Sallah S, Wan JY, Nguyen NP. Venous thrombosis in patients with solid tumors: determination of frequency and characteristics. Thromb Haemost 2002;87:575–9.

[144] Thodiyil PA, Kakkar AK. Variation in relative risk of venous thromboembolism in different cancers. Thromb Haemost 2002;87:1076–7.

[145] Kakkar AK, Haas S, Walsh D, et al. Prevention of perioperative venous thromboembolism: outcome after cancer and non-cancer surgery. [abstract]. Thromb Haemost 2001; 86(Suppl):OC1732.

[146] Rajan R, Gafni A, Levine M, et al. Very low-dose warfarin prophylaxis to prevent thromboembolism in women with metastatic breast cancer receiving chemotherapy: an economic evaluation. J Clin Oncol 1995;13:42–6.

[147] Attia J, Ray JG, Cook DJ, et al. Deep vein thrombosis and its prevention in critically ill adults. Arch Intern Med 2001;161:1268–79.

[148] Geerts W, Cook D, Selby R, et al. Venous thromboembolism and its prevention in critical care. J Crit Care 2002;17:95–104.

[149] Dorffler-Melly J, de Jonge E, de Pont AC, et al. Bioavailability of subcutaneous low-molecular-weight heparin to patients on vasopressors. Lancet 2002;359:849–50.

[150] Liska WD, Poteet BA. Pulmonary embolism associated with canine total hip replacement. Vet Surg 2003;32(2):178–86.

[151] Feldman EC, Nelson RW. Canine hyperadrenocorticism (Cushing's syndrome). In: Feldman EC, Nelson RW, editors. Canine and feline endocrinology and reproduction. St Louis: WB Saunders; 2004. p. 252–352.

[152] Gregory CR, Kyles AE, Bernsteen L, et al. Results of clinical renal transplantation in 15 dogs using triple drug immunosuppressive therapy. Vet Surg 2006;35(2):105–12.

[153] La Rue MJ, Murtaugh RJ. Pulmonary thromboembolism in dogs: 47 cases (1986–1987). J Am Vet Med Assoc 1990;197(10):1368–72.

[154] Johnson LR, Lappin MR, Baker DC. Pulmonary thromboembolism in 29 dogs: 1985–1995. J Vet Intern Med 1999;13(4):338–45.

[155] Schermerhorn T. Pulmonary thromboembolism in cats. J Vet Intern Med 2004;18(4): 533–5.

[156] Baines EA. Gross pulmonary thrombosis in a greyhound. J Small Anim Pract 2001;42(9): 448–53.

[157] Palmer KG. Clinical manifestations and associated disease syndromes in dogs with cranial vena cava thrombosis: 17 cases (1989–1996). J Am Vet Med Assoc 1998;213(2):220–4.

[158] Ritt MG. Nephrotic syndrome resulting in thromboembolic disease and disseminated intravascular coagulation in a dog. J Am Anim Hosp Assoc 1997;33(5):385–91.

[159] Carter AJ. Aortic thrombosis in a dog with glomerulonephritis. J S Afr Vet Assoc 1994; 65(4):189–92.

[160] Stone MS. Lupus-type "anticoagulant" in a dog with hemolysis and thrombosis. J Vet Intern Med 1994;8(1):57–61.

[161] Green RA. Hypercoagulable state in three dogs with nephrotic syndrome: role of acquired antithrombin III deficiency. J Am Vet Med Assoc 2004;18(4):533–5.

[162] Cook AK, Cowgill LD. Clinical and pathological features of protein-losing glomerular disease in the dog: a review of 137 cases (1985–1992). J Am Anim Hosp Assoc 1996;32: 313–22.

[163] Carr AP, Panciera DL, Kidd L. Prognostic factors for mortality and thromboembolism in canine immune-mediated hemolytic anemia: a retrospective study of 72 dogs. J Vet Intern Med 2002;16(5):504–9.

[164] Tilley LP, Liu SK, Gilbertson SR, et al. Primary myocardial disease in the cat. A model for human cardiomyopathy. Am J Pathol 1977;86:493–522.

[165] Grauer GF. CVT update: canine glomerulonephritis. In: Bonagura JD, editor. Kirk's current veterinary therapy XIII. Philadelphia: WB Saunders Co; 2000. p. 851–3.

[166] Abdullah R. Hemostatic abnormalities in nephrotic syndrome. Vet Clin North Am Small Anim Pract 1988;18(1):105–13.

[167] Rasedee A, Feldman BF. Nephrotic syndrome: a platelet hyperaggregability state. Vet Res Commun 1985;9:199–211.

[168] Littman MP, Dambach DM, Vaden SL, et al. Familial protein-enteropathy and protein-losing nephropathy in soft coated wheaten terriers: 222 cases (1983–1997). J Vet Intern Med 2000;14:68–80.

[169] Otto CM, Reiser TM, Brooks MB, et al. Evidence of hypercoagulability in dogs with parvoviral enteritis. J Am Vet Med Assoc 2000;217(10):1500–4.

[170] Nichols R. Complications and concurrent disease associated with canine hyperadrenocorticism. Vet Clin North Am Small Anim Pract 1997;27(2):309–19.

[171] Scott-Moncreiff JC, Treadwell NG, McCullough SM, et al. Hemostatic abnormalities in dogs with primary immune-mediated anemia. J Am Anim Hosp Assoc 2001;37:220–7.

[172] Klein MK, Dow SW, Rosychuck RAW. Pulmonary thromboembolism associated with immune-mediated hemolytic anemia in dogs: ten cases (1982–1987). J Am Vet Med Assoc 1989;195:246–50.

[173] McManus PM, Craig LE. Correlation between leukocytosis and necropsy findings in dogs with immune-mediated hemolytic anemia: 34 cases (1994–1999). J Am Vet Med Assoc 2001;218:1308–13.

[174] Weinkle TK, Center SA, Randolf JF, et al. Evaluation of prognostic factors, survival rates, and treatment protocols for immune-mediated hemolytic anemia in dogs: 151 cases (1993-2002). J Am Vet Med Assoc 2005;226(11):1869–80.

[175] Slappendel RJ. Disseminated intravascular coagulation. Vet Clin North Am Small Anim Pract 1988;18(1):169–84.

[176] Owen CA, Bowie EJW. Effect of heparin on chronically induced intravascular coagulation in dogs. Am J Physiol 1975;229–49.

[177] Mant MJ, King EG. Severe, acute disseminated intravascular coagulation. A reappraisal of its pathophysiology, clinical significance and therapy, based on 47 patients. Am J Med 1979;67(4):557–63.

[178] Mischke R, Fehr M, Nolte I. Efficacy of low molecular weight heparin in a canine model of thromboplastin-induced disseminated intravascular coagulation. Res Vet Sci 2005;79(1): 69–76.

[179] O'Keefe DA, Couto G. Coagulation abnormalities associated with neoplasia. Vet Clin North Am Small Anim Pract 1988;18(1):157–67.

Vet Clin Small Anim 37 (2007) 611–616

VETERINARY CLINICS
SMALL ANIMAL PRACTICE

INDEX

0195-5616/07/$ – see front matter
doi:10.1016/S0195-5616(07)00047-2

Moving?

Make sure your subscription moves with you!

To notify us of your new address, find your **Clinics Account Number** (located on your mailing label above your name), and contact customer service at:

E-mail: elspcs@elsevier.com

800-654-2452 (subscribers in the U.S. & Canada)
407-345-4000 (subscribers outside of the U.S. & Canada)

Fax number: 407-363-9661

Elsevier Periodicals Customer Service
6277 Sea Harbor Drive
Orlando, FL 32887-4800

*To ensure uninterrupted delivery of your subscription, please notify us at least 4 weeks in advance of move.

ELSEVIER